THE
ICU QUICK
REFERENCE

Sheree Comer, R.N., M.S., C.C.R.N.

A SKIDMORE-ROTH PUBLICATION

PUBLISHING

Publisher: Linda Skidmore-Roth
Cover design: Martha A. Romero
Developmental Editor: Alexandra Swann

Copyright © 1994 by Skidmore-Roth Publishing, Inc. All rights reserved. No part of this book may be copied or transmitted in any form or by any means without written permission from the publisher.

Notice: The author and publisher of this volume have taken care to make certain that all information is correct and compatible with standards generally accepted at the time of publication. Because the science of nursing is constantly changing and expanding, new techniques and concepts are continually implemented. Therefore, the reader is encouraged to stay abreast of new developments in the nursing field and to be aware that policies vary according to the guidelines of each school or institution.

Comer, Sheree Raye
The ICU Quick Reference

ISBN 1-56930-003-8
1. Nursing Handbooks, Manuals
2. Medical Handbooks, Manuals

SKIDMORE-ROTH PUBLISHING, INC.
7730 Trade Center Ave.
El Paso, Texas 79912
1 (800)825-3150

TABLE OF CONTENTS

LABORATORY VALUES
Normal Laboratory Values 3
Anion Gap 30
DIC Profile Lab 31
White Blood Cell Differential 32
Laboratory Results for Specific
Diseases 33
Microscopic Examination of Urine 34
Routine Urinalysis 38
Laboratory Findings Suggestive of
Medical Disorders 39
Colloid Oncotic Pressure 49
Serum Osmolality 49
Platelets 49
Routine Urinalysis 50
Effects of Drugs on Routine Urinalysis 52
Cerebrospinal Fluid Lab Values 56

MEDICATIONS AND MEDICATION CHARTS
Commonly-used Medications 59
Apresoline Drip Chart 212
Tridil Table 213
Starting Rates for Vasoactive Drugs 214
Method for Rapid Calculation of IV Drips 215
Inocor Chart 218
Nipride Chart 219
Dobutamine Chart 224
Dopamine Chart 226
Children's Dopamine Chart 229
Children's Dobutrex Chart 231

ii *Table of Contents*

Cardiovascular Drugs 232

ALGORITHMS

Adult Emergency Cardiac Care Algorithm 233
Ventricular Fibrillation/Pulseless
Ventricular Tachycardia Algorithm 235
Pulseless Electrical Activity or
Electromechanical Dissociation Algorithm 238
Asystole Algorithm 240
Bradycardia Algorithm 242
Electrical Cardioversion Algorithm 244
Hemodynamic Algorithm 245
Acute MI/CP Algorithm 246
Hypotension, Shock, and Acute Pulmonary
Edema Algorithm 247
Tachycardia Algorithm 250

HEMODYNAMIC MONITORING

Preload 255
Afterload 256
Autonomic Nervous System 256
Formulas and Normals for
Hemodynamic Parameters 258
Body Surface Area Chart 260
Fick Method of ComputingCardiac Output 261
PA Catheter Waveforms 263
Left Atrial Lines 264
Right Atrial Pressure Waveforms 265
Clinical Symptoms of Various
Types of Shock States 267
Symptoms of Cardiac Tamponade 269
Comparing Shock's Three Stages 270

The ICU Quick Reference iii

Continuous Mixed Venous Oxygen
  Saturation Monitoring 275
Pulmonary Artery Catheters 276
Troubleshooting a PA Monitor 279

CARDIAC MONITORING AND PACEMAKERS
Leads 286
Modified Chest Lead 287
Probability of SVT vs. VT 288
QRS Complexes 290
EKG Wave Patterns 291
Heart Rate Calculation 293
EKG Rhythm Determination 294
Dangerous Premature Ventricular Contractions 295
Normals on 12-Lead EKG 295
EKG Rhythm Determination 296
Heart Murmurs and Conditions that Cause Them .. 301
Einthoven's Triangle 303
Axis Determination 304
EKG Changes 305
EKG Changes in Myocardial Infarction 306
Causes of Hypertrophy 309
AV Conduction Defects 309
EKG Data and Changes With Certain Conditions .. 310
Events in the Cardiac Cycle 314
Basic Parts of a Pacemaker 315
Pacemaker Rates 317
Pacemaker Terminology 317
Pacemakers 324
Troubleshooting Pacemakers 326
Auscultation of Heart Sounds 328

iv *Table of Contents*

Procedure for Immediate Return of
Post-op Cardiac Patient 330
Intra-Aortic Balloon Therapy 333
IABP Terminology 335
IABP Waveform 339
Symptoms of Cardiac Tamponade 340
Cardiac Catheterization Complications 341
Percutaneous Transluminal Coronary
Angioplasty Complications 341
Causes of Coronary Artery Reocclusion
after PTCA 342
Wolff-Parkinson-White Syndrome 342
Wellen's Syndrome 343

RESPIRATORY CARE
Oxygen Delivery Systems 347
Causes of Inadequate Alveolar
Ventilation 347
Causes of Decreased Diffusion 348
Causes of Decreased Oxygen Transport 348
Pulmonary Terminology 349
Determining Problems With Ventilators 350
Hazards of Oxygen Therapy 351
Oxygen Toxicity 352
Formulas and Normals for Respiratory
Equations 352
Indications for Mechanical Ventilation 354
Problems Associated with Mechanical
Ventilation 355

The ICU Quick Reference v

Ventilator Modes 355
Peep 357
Guide to Initial Settings of Ventilators 359
Indications for Weaning From Ventilator 360
Determining ABG Results 361
Continuous Mixed Venous Oxygen
Saturation Monitoring 362
Normals For Mixed Venous Blood Gases 363
Common Causes and Treatment for Acid
Base Disorders 363
Breath Sounds 365
Oxygen Dissociation Curve 367
Comparison of Bronchitis Versus Emphysema 368
Ventilation Perfusion Scans 368
Adult Respiratory Distress Syndrome 369
ARDS Physiology 370

RENAL AND ENDOCRINE SYSTEMS
Electrolyte and Mineral Imbalances/Causes 373
Daily Approximate Requirements 376
Common Signs and Symptoms of Endocrine
Dysfunction 376
The Renin-Angiotensin Aldosterone Feedback
System 379
Fluid and Electrolyte Imbalances 380
Endocrine System Glands and Hormones
Secreted 388
Endocrine Problems 389
Syndrome of Inappropriate Antidiuretic
Hormone 392
Differences Between Prerenal, Renal,
and Postrenal Failure 394

vi *Table of Contents*

Glomerular Filtration Rate 395

NEUROLOGIC SYSTEM
Glasgow Coma Scale 399
Initial Management of Head Injury Patients 400
Pupillary Size 400
Pediatric Coma Scale 401
Best Verbal Response 402
Neurologic Problems 403
Grading Systems of Deep Tendon Reflexes 406
Cranial Nerves 407
Autonomic Nervous System Reactions 408

PEDIATRICS
Physiologically Unstable Infants 411
Cardiopulmonary Assessment 412
Signs and Symptoms of Deterioration 413
Dysrhythmias in Children 415
Approximate Children's Dosages 417
Basic Life Support in Children 418
Information for Pediatric Emergency
Medications 424
Maintenance Calories 427
Calculation of Drug Dosages 427
Determining Drug Administration Rates with
Variable Drug Concentrations 428
Modification of Maintenance Fluid
Requirements Based on Condition 430
Congenital Heart Defects 433

The ICU Quick Reference vii

WEIGHTS AND MEASURES

Temperature Equivalents 441
Frequently Used Equivalents in the Metric System . 443
Standard Basal Calories 445
Abdominal Anatomic Sites 446
Clotting Factors and Their Synonyms 447
Symptoms and Possible Poisons 448
Miscellaneous Signs and Symptoms 461
Blood Type Compatibility 470
What to Chart 471

Appendix: Glossary of Abbreviations 475

References 484

Index 487

LABORATORY VALUES

2 Laboratory Values

TABLE OF CONTENTS

Normal Laboratory Values 3
Anion Gap 30
DIC Profile Lab 31
White Blood Cell Differential 32
Laboratory Results for Specific
Diseases 33
Microscopic Examination of Urine 34
Routine Urinalysis 38
Laboratory Findings Suggestive of
Medical Disorders 39
Colloid Oncotic Pressure 49
Serum Osmolality 49
Platelets 49
Routine Urinalysis 50
Effects of Drugs on Routine Urinalysis 52
Cerebrospinal Fluid Lab Values 56

NORMAL LABORATORY VALUES

Acetaminophen Level *(Tylenol)* Therapeutic range Adult and child	5-20 µg/ml 31-124 µmol/L(SI)
Toxic level Hepatic toxicity Adult Child	50 µm/ml 200 mg/ml 305 µmol/L (SI) 140 mg/kg
Activated Coagulation Time (ACT)	90-120 secs
Acid Phosphatase Adult Child Newborn	0-0.8 IU/L 0.13-0.63 U/L (SI) 0.5-11 U/ml 8.6-12.6 U/L 10.3-16.3 U/ml
A/G Ratio	1.0-2.2

4 Laboratory Values

NORMAL LABORATORY VALUES

Alanine Aminotransferase (ALT) Adult Child Newborn	4-45 IU/L 4-35 U/L (SI) Same as adult 4 Times adult level
Albumin, Serum Adult Child Infant Newborn	3.0-5.5 gm/dl 32-45 gm/L(SI) 4.0-5.8 gm/dl 4.4-5.4 gm/dl 2.9-5.4 gm/dl
Alkaline Phosphatase Adult Child Infant	30-115 IU/L 20-90 IU/L (SI) 30-85 Im U/ml May be 3 times adult levels 85-210 Im U/ml
Alpha-1 Antitrypsin Adult Age 6 weeks to 18 yrs Newborn	> 250 mg/dl 85-213 mg/dl 147-200 mg/dl
Alpha-2 Macroglobulin	146-369 ng/dl 0.5-1.0 gm/dl

NORMAL LABORATORY VALUES

Amino Acid Screen, Urine	Negative
Ammonia, Plasma Adult Child Newborn	10-40 mg/dl 11-35 µmol/L (SI) 15-110 µg/dl 40-80 mg/dl 90-145 mg/dl
Amylase, Serum Adult Child	80-150 Somogyi U/dl 20-110 IU/L 80-180 U/dl 110-300 U/L (SI)
Amylase, Urine	5000 Somogyi U/24 hrs 260-950 U/24 hrs 4-37 IU/2hrs 24-76 U/ml 6.1-48.0 U/L (SI)
Anti-DNase B Titer Preschool School Age Adult	1:60 1:170 1:85
Antinuclear Antibody Titer (ANA)	Negative < 1:70 generally rules out autoimmune disease

NORMAL LABORATORY VALUES

Anti-Smooth Muscle Antibody (ASMA)	Negative No titers at > 1:20
Anti-Strep Screen	Negative
Anti-Strep Titer	< 4-fold rise ≤ 160 Todd U/ml
Anti-Thrombin III Assay	80-120% 22-39 mg/dl
Aspartate Aminotransferase (AST) Adult Child Newborn	 4-36 IU/L 8-35 U/L (SI) Same as adult 15-60 U/L
Bence Jones Protein	Negative
Bicarbonate Venous Adult Arterial Adult Newborn	 19-25 mEq/L 22-26 mEq/L 16-24 mEq/L

NORMAL LABORATORY VALUES

Bilirubin, Direct, Serum Adult Child Newborn	0.1-0.3 mg/dl 1.7-5.1 µmol/L (SI) 0.2-0.8 mg/dl 0-6 mg/dl 17-205 µmol/L(SI)
Bilirubin, Fecal	Negative
Bilirubin, Indirect, Serum	0.2-8.0 mg/dl < 18 µmol/L (SI)
Bilirubin, Micro	0.2-1.2 mg/dl
Bilirubin, Total Adult Newborn	0.1-1.0 mg/dl 1.8-21 micromoles/L (SI) 1-12 mg/dl
Bilirubin, Urine	Negative: 0.02 mg/dl
Bleeding Time Template IVY Duke	2-8 minutes 1-9 minutes 1-3 minutes

8 Laboratory Values

NORMAL LABORATORY VALUES

Blood Urea Nitrogen (BUN)	
Adult	10-20 mg/dl
	3-8 mmol/L (SI)
Child	5-20 mg/dl
Infant	5-15 mg/dl
Newborn	3-12 mg/dl
Calcium, Serum	
Adult	8.5-10.5 mg dl
	2.3-2.8 mmol/L(SI)
Child	8-11.5 mg/dl
Infant	9-12 mg/dl
Newborn	9.0-10.6 mg/dl
Calcium, Urine	100-300 mg/24 hrs
	< 6.3 mmol/d (SI)
Calcium Urine Screen	Negative
Carbon Dioxide (CO_2)	22-34 mEq/L
	22-34 mmol/L (SI)
Carbamazepine Level (Tegretol)	
Therapeutic range	5-12 μg/ml
Toxic Level	> 12 μg/ml

NORMAL LABORATORY VALUES

Ceruloplasmin Adult Newborn	17-34 mg/dl Low Level
Chloride, Serum Adult Child Newborn	96-106 mEq/L 96-106 mmol/L (SI) 90-110 mEq/L 90-110 mmol/L (SI) 95-110 mEq/L 95-110 mmol/L (SI)
Chloride, Urine	110-250 mEq/L
Cholesterol Adult < 40 years Adult > 40 years Child Infant	120-200 mg/dl 150-230 mg/dl 3.0-6.5 mmol/L (SI) 120-250 mg/dl 70-175 mg/dl
Cholesterol, HDL Low coronary risk Intermediate coronary risk High coronary risk	> 45 mg/dl 35-55 mg/dl < 35 mg/dl
Cold Agglutinins	Negative; < 1:16, may be higher in elderly

Laboratory Values

NORMAL LABORATORY VALUES

Complement, (C-3)	83-177 mg/dl 0.88-1.80 gm/L (SI)
Complement, (C-4)	15-45 mg/dl 0.12-0.45 gm/L (SI)
Complement, Total	56-150 U/ml 41-90 Hemo U
Complete Blood Count (CBC) *Red blood cell count (RBC)* Male Female Child Infant Newborn	 $4.7\text{-}6.1 \times 10^6$/cu mm $4.2\text{-}5.4 \times 10^6$/cu mm $3.8\text{-}5.4 \times 10^6$/cu mm $3.8\text{-}5.5 \times 10^6$/cu mm $4.4\text{-}5.8 \times 10^6$/cu mm
White blood cell count (WBC) Adult Child Infant Newborn	 $4.5\text{-}10.5 \times 1000$/cu mm $4.5\text{-}10.5 \times 10^9$/L (SI) $6\text{-}17 \times 1000$/cu mm $9\text{-}30 \times 1000$/cu mm $7\text{-}35 \times 1000$/cu mm

NORMAL LABORATORY VALUES

Differential White Cell Count	Adults	Children
Polys	40-70%	38-77%
Bands	0-5%	0-6%
Eosinophils	1-3%	1-8%
Basophils	0-2%	0.3-1.4%
Lymphocytes	25-45%	16-51%
Reactive lymphocytes	6%	0-6%
Monocytes	1-10%	1-12%

Hemoglobin (HMG)	
Male	130-175 gm/L (SI)
	13.0-17.5 gm/dl
Female	115-160 gm/L (SI)
	11.5-16.0 gm/dl
Child	11/16 gm/dl
	110-160 gm/L (SI)
Infant	10-14 gm/dl
	100-140 gm/L (SI)
Newborn	14-24 gm/dl
	140-240 gm/L (SI)

NORMAL LABORATORY VALUES

Hematocrit (HCT)	
Male	0.42-0.52 (SI) 42-52%
Female	38-46 (SI) 38-46%
Child	0.30-0.44 (SI) 30-44%
Infant	0.30-0.40 (SI) 30-40%
Newborn	0.45-0.65 (SI) 45-65%
Mean Corpuscular Hemoglobin (MCH) = $\frac{HMG}{RBC}$	
Adult and Child	26-34 pg/red cell
Newborn	32-34 pg/red cell
Mean Corpuscular Hemoglobin Concentration (MCHC) = $\frac{HMG}{HCT}$	
Adult and Child	31-37%
Newborn	32-33 %
Mean Corpuscular Volume (MCV) = $\frac{HCT}{RBC}$	80-100 cubic microns/red cell

NORMAL LABORATORY VALUES

Red Cell Distribution Width (RDW)	11-15%
Platelet count	150-450 × 10³ cu mm
Creatine Phosphokinase (CPK, CK)	12-70 U/ml 5-45 IU/L 0.08-0.58 μmol/L
Male Female Infants Newborn	25-175 IU/L 25-145 IU/L 10-55 U/ml 4 times adult levels 68-580 U/L
CPK Isoenzymes CPK-BB CPK-MB CPK-MM	 0 0-8 IU/L 5-70 IU/L
Creatinine Clearance Male Female Elderly Newborn	 130-170 ml/min 75-115 ml/min decrease by 6 ml/min/decade 40-65 ml/min

NORMAL LABORATORY VALUES

Creatinine, Serum Adult Child Newborn	0.7-1.5 mg/dl 58-106 μmol/L (SI) 0.3-0.7 mg/dl 44-106 μmol/L 0.3-1.2 mg/dl
Creatinine, Urine Male Female	1000-2000 mg/24 hrs 9-17 mmol/24 hrs (SI) 800-1100 mg/24 hrs 7-15 mmol/24 hrs (SI)
C-Reactive Protein, Quantitative	Negative or < 0.6 mg/dl
Digoxin Therapeutic range: Adult Child Infant Toxic Level: Adult Infant	 0.6-2 ng/ml 0.6-2 nmol/L (SI) Same as adult 1-3 ng/ml > 2 ng/ml > 3.5 ng/ml

NORMAL LABORATORY VALUES

Dilantin Level (Phenytoin) Therapeutic range Toxic level Adult Child	10-20 µ/ml 40-80 µmol/L (SI) > 30 µg/ml > 79.2 µmol/L (SI) > 15-20 µg/ml > 55-78 µ mol/L (SI)
Eosinophil Count	0-450/cu mm 1-4%
Erythrocyte Sedimentation Rate (ESR) Adult Child	 0-20 mm/hr 0-14 mm/hr
Estriol	Varies according to weeks of gestation and from day to day in same patient
Euglobulin Clot Lysis	2-4 hrs
Fat, Fecal, Qualitative	Small amount of neutral fat
Fat, Fecal, Quantitative	1-7 gm/24 hrs as fatty acids
Febrile Agglutinins	Negative ≤ 1:80

16 Laboratory Values

NORMAL LABORATORY VALUES

Fibrin Split Products (FSP)	Up to 10 µg/ml
Fibrinogen Adult Child Newborn	 180-400 mg/dl 68-4 mg/dl (SI) Same as adult 150-300 mg/dl
Folic Acid	5-25 ng/ml 11-56 nmol/L (SI)
Gamma Glutamyl Transferase (GGT)	6-37 U/L 5-40 IU/L (SI)
Gentamicin Levels Peak Therapeutic Toxic Trough Therapeutic Toxic	 5-10 µg/ml > 12 µg/ml 1-2 µg/ml > 2 µg/ml
Globulin, Serum Total	 2.4-3.5 gm/dl

NORMAL LABORATORY VALUES

Globulin Alpha 1 Alpha 2 Beta Gamma	0.1-0.4 gm/dl 0.5-1 gm/dl 0.7-1.2 gm/dl 0.5-1.6 gm/dl
Glucose, CSF	40-70 mg/dl ⅔ of blood glucose
Glucose, Serum, fasting Adult < 50 years Adult > 50 years	70-115 mg/dl 80-125 mg/dl 3.8-6 mmol/L (SI)
Child Newborn	60-100 mg/dl 30-80 mg/dl
Glucose urine	Negative
Glycosylated Hemoglobin (HbA_{1c})	2.2-4.8 % 3.5-6.1 % of total Hmg
Ham's Test	No hemolysis
Haptoglobin	26-185 mg/dl

Laboratory Values

NORMAL LABORATORY VALUES

Hemoglobin F Adult Neonate	< 2% 50-90%
Hemosiderin	Negative
Herpes I and II Immunofluorescence Titer	< 1:100
5-Hydroxyindolacetic Acid (5HIAA)	2.8-8 mg/24 hrs 3-10 mg/24 hrs
Hemocystine	Negative
17-Hydroxycorticosteroids (17-OHCS) Male Female Child	 4-13 mg/24 hrs 3-12 mg/24 hrs 1.5-4.5 mg/24 hrs
Immunoglobulin A, (IgA) Adult Child Infant Newborn	 85-385 mg/dl 20-200 mg/dl 10-90 mg/dl 0-11 mg/dl

NORMAL LABORATORY VALUES

Immunoglobulin E, (IgE) Adult	0-104 mg/dl
Immunoglobulin G, (IgG) Adult Child Infant Newborn	565-1765 mg/dl 650-1300 mg/dl 200-1100 mg/dl 650-1250 mg/dl
Immunoglobulin M, (IgM) Adult Child Infant Newborn	55-375 mg/dl 50-375 mg/dl 30-120 mg/dl 10-80 mg/dl 5-35 mg/dl
Immunoglobulin G, CSF	< 12% of total protein
Iron Adult Child Newborn	60-190 mg/dl 10-25 µmol/dl (SI) 40-100 gm/dl 100-200 gm/dl

NORMAL LABORATORY VALUES

Iron-binding capacity (TIBC) Adult Child Newborn	250-400 mg/dl 54-64 µmol/L (SI) 100-350 gm/dl 60-170 gm/dl
17 Ketogenic Steroids (17 KGS) Male Female	5-23 mg/24 hrs 3-15 mg/24 hrs
Ketones, Urine	Negative
17 Ketosteroids (17-KS) Male adult Male adolescent Female adult Female adolescent	8-15 mg/24hrs 3-18 mg/24 hrs 6-12 mg/24 hrs 3-12 mg/24 hrs
Lactic Acid, Serum	0.6-2.2 mEq/L 6-22 mg/dl

NORMAL LABORATORY VALUES

Lactic Dehydrogenase (LDH)	
Adult	60-225 IU/L
	30-62 U/L (SI)
Child	50-150 IU/L
	60-170 U/L
Newborn	300-1600 IU/L
	160-450 U/L
LDH Isoenzymes	
LDH1	18-27 %
	0.18-0.27 (SI)
LDH2	28-38%
	0.28-0.38 (SI)
LDH3	18-26%
	0.18-0.26 (SI)
LDH4	4-9%
	0.04-0.09 (SI)
LDH5	0-5%
	0-0.05 (SI)
LE Prep	Negative
Lee-White Clotting Time	6-12 mins
Lidocaine Level	
Therapeutic range	1.1-5.6 µg/ml
	5.0-23.4 mol/L (SI)
Toxic Level	> 6 µg/ml

NORMAL LABORATORY VALUES

Lipase, Serum	< 1.0 U/ml 5-150 IU/L
Lithium Level Therapeutic range Toxic level Fatal level	0.5-1.5 meq/L 0.5-1.5 µmol/L > 2.0 meq/L > 4.0 meq/L
Magnesium, Serum Adult Child	1.5-2.0 meq/L 0.7-1.1 mmol/L (SI) 1.7-2.2 meq/L
Microsomal Antibody Titer	< 1:00
Monotest	Negative
Nitroblue Tetrazolium Titer (NBT)	< 10% NBT positive neutrophils
Occult Blood, Fecal	Negative
Occult Blood, Urine	Negative
Orosomucoid	30-135 mg/dl
Osmolality, Serum	280-295 mOsm/kg 280-295 mmol/L (SI)

NORMAL LABORATORY VALUES

Osmolality, Urine	
Adult	38-1400 mmol /kg/H_2O
	200-800 mOsm/kg/H_2O
	200-800 mmol/kg (SI)
Child	Same as adult
Newborn	100-550 mOsm/kg/H_2O
	100-550 mmol/kg (SI)
Osmotic Fragility	
Initial hemolysis	0.44 ± 0.02% NaCl
Complete hemolysis	0.32 ± 0.02% NaCl
Ox-Cell Hemolysis Titer	< 1:56 titer
pH, Urine	Approximately 6.0
Partial Thromboplastin Time (PTT)	0-35 secs
Phenobarbital Level	
Therapeutic range	15-30 µg/ml
Toxic level	> 40 µg/ml

NORMAL LABORATORY VALUES

Phenytoin Level (Dilantin) Therapeutic range	1.0-2.0 mg/dl 10-20 μg/ml 40-80 μmol/L (SI)
Toxic level Adult	> 20 μg/ml > 79.2 μmol/L (SI)
Child	> 15-20 μmol/L (SI) 55-78 μmol/L (SI)
Phosphorus, Serum Adult	2.5-4.6 mg/dl 0.8-1.5 mmol/L (SI)
Child	2.4-4.1 mEq/L 1.29-2.26 mmol/L (SI)
Newborn	2.4-5.9 mEq/L 1.4-3.0 mmol/L (SI)
Phosphorus, Urine	900-1300 mg/24 hrs
Plasma Hemoglobin	< 3 mg/dl
Plasminogen	80-120%
Platelet Count	150-450 × 1000/cu mm 150-450 × 10^6/L

NORMAL LABORATORY VALUES

Potassium, Serum Adult	3.5-5.5 mEq/L 3.5-5.5 mmol/L (SI)
Child	3.5-4.7 mEq/L
Newborn	3.9-5.9 mEq/L
Potassium, Urine	25-100 mEq/24 hrs
Prealbumin	11-33 mg/dl
Procainamide Level Therapeutic range Toxic level N-acetyl-procainamide (NAPA) Therapeutic range Toxic level	4-10 µ/ml > 12 µg/ml 2-8 µg/ml >30 µg/ml
Protein, Total, Serum Adult	6.6-7.9 gm/dl 6-8 gm/L (SI)
Child	6.2-8.0 gm/dl
Newborn	4.5-7.5 gm/dl
Protein, Total, Urine	10-100 mg/24 hrs
Prothrombin Time (PT)	11-12.5 secs

Normal Laboratory Values

Pseudocholinesterase	7-14 IU/ml 1900-3800 U/L
Rheumatoid Factor (RA)	Negative < 1:20
Quinidine Level Therapeutic range Toxic level	2.3-5.0 µg/ml > 10 µg/ml
Reducing Substances, Fecal and Urine	Negative
Respiratory Syncytial Virus Antibodies (RSV)	< 1:8 Titer
Reticulocyte Count Adult Child Newborn	25,000-75,000 mm^3 0.5-1.5% 25-75 × 10^9/L (SI) 0.5-2% of all RBCS 2-6% of all RBCs
Salicylate level Therapeutic range Toxic level Adult Child	100-200 µg/ml 2-29 mg/dl (minor) > 30 mg/dl (major) > 50 mg/dl

NORMAL LABORATORY VALUES

Sedimentation Rate (Westergren Method) Male Female Child (1-14 years) Newborn	0-15 mm/hr (SI) 0-20 mm/hr (SI) 0-15 mm/hr 0-2 mm/hr
Syphilis, (Serological Test) (RPR)	Non-reactive
Serotonin, 5HIAA, Quantitative	2-4 mg/24 hrs 2.8-8.0 mg/24 hrs
SGOT Adult Child Newborn	4-36 IU/L 8-35 U/L (SI) Same as adult 4 times adult level
SGPT Adult Child Newborn	4-45 IU/L 4-35 U/L (SI) Same as adult 15-60 U/L

NORMAL LABORATORY VALUES

Sodium, Serum	
Adult	134-147 mEq/L
	134-147 mmol/L(SI)
Child	138-145 mEq/L
	138-145 mmol/L (SI)
Newborn	126-166 mEq/L
	126-166 mmol/L (SI)
Sodium, Urine	100-260 mEq/24 hrs
Specific Gravity, Urine	
Adult	1.005-1.030
Child	1:005-1.030
Newborn	1.001-1.020
Sugar Water Test	No hemolysis
Sweat Chloride	
Adult	< 60 mEq/L
	4-60 mmol/L (SI)
Child	< 50 mEq/L
Theophylline level	
Therapeutic range	10-20 µg/ml
Toxic level	26-110 mol/L (SI)
Adult	> 20 µg/ml
	> 110 mol/L (SI)
Child	Same as adult
Infant	8-10 µg/ml

NORMAL LABORATORY VALUES

Thrombin Clotting Time	8-10 secs
Thromboplastin	20-30 secs
Thyroid-Stimulating Hormone (TSH) Adult Child/Newborn	2-10 U/ml 2.5-5 IU/ml > 10^{-3} IU/L (SI) < 3 ng/ml 3-18 U/ml < 251 IU/ml by 3rd day or life
Tobramycin Level Peak therapeutic range Peak toxic level Trough therapeutic range Trough toxic level	5-10 µg/ml > 12 µg/ml < 2 µg/ml > 2 µg/ml 204-360 mg/dl
Transferrin	170-340 mg/dl
Triglycerides Adult Child Infant	10-190 mg/dl 0.11-2.11 mmol/L (SI) 36-138 mg/dl 30-86 mg/dl

Laboratory Values

NORMAL LABORATORY VALUES	
Uric Acid Male Female Child	2.1-8.5 mg/dl 0.24-0.5 mmol/L (SI) 2.2.-6.6 mg/dl 0.16-0.4 mmol/L (SI) 2.5-8 mg/dl
Vanillylmandelic Acid (VMA) Adult Newborn	0.5-12.0 mg/ 24 hrs 2-7 mg/24 hrs < 1.0 mg/24 hrs

THE ANION GAP (AGAP)

- Anion gap = $(Na^+ + K^+) - (Cl^- + HCO_3^-)$ [or serum CO_2]
- Normal usually 8 to 12 mEq/L
- A high anion gap means that new acid is being formed; if anion gap is present, the patient is losing HCO_3^- ion.
- If Agap is increased, this means that hydrogen ion has been added to the extra-cellular fluid with some anion other than chloride.$^+$
- If Agap is not increased the reduction of HCO_3^- has resulted from a loss of HCO_3^- or addition of H^+ with CL^-.

Low Agap (< 6 mEq/L)
- Hypoalbuminemia
- Metabolic acidosis
- Hyperviscosity
- Hypermagnesemia
- Severe hypernatremia
- Lactic acidosis
- Hypercalcemia
- Lithium toxicity
- Multiple myeloma

High Agap (> 12 mEq/L)
Metabolic acidosis with concurrent high Agap—(a decrease in HCO_3^- matched by an equal increase in non-chloride anion)
- Hyperalbuminemia
- High-dose PCN antibiotics
- Lactic acidosis
- Hemodialysis
- Alkalosis
- DKA

Normal Agap
- 8-12 mEq/L
- Metabolic acidosis with normal Agap

DIC PROFILE LAB

- Protime [normal 11 to 13 seconds] prolonged
- Platelet count [normal 150 to 400 thousand] decreased
- APTT [normal 20 to 30 seconds] prolonged
- Fibrinogen [normal 200 to 400] decreased
- Fibrin split products [normal less than 10] elevated; usually > 40 when severe
- Red Cell Distribution Width (RDW) [normal 11-15] slightly to significantly increased
- D-Dimer (similar to fibrin split products) elevated

Beth Minssen, R.N., M.A., C.C.R.N., Understanding Lab, 2nd edition, Used by permission of the author

WHITE BLOOD CELL DIFFERENTIAL

- Neutrophils (polys, segs) [normal 39-79% of total WBC count].
- Neutrophils, immature (bands) (bands greater than 5 are significant for acute infection—referred to as a "shift to the left").
- If metacytes or myelocytes are present, patient has an acute bacterial infection.
- Eosinophils [normal 0-5% of total WBC count]—elevated amounts are seen in allergic conditions and with parasitic diseases.
- Basophils [normal 0-2% of total WBC count]—the element that helps release heparin and histamine at the site in the inflammatory response.
- Lymphocytes (B-lymphocytes provide humoral immunity, antibodies T-lymphocytes orchestrate antibody and complement activity leading to increased chemotaxis and permeability).
- Monocytes [normal 3-8 % of total WBC count]—elevated amounts are seen in chronic infections. When these leave the blood stream and attach to tissues, they are then known as issue macrophages. Stationary monocytes are known as histiocytes.

Beth Minssen, R.N., M.A., C.C.R.N, Understanding Lab, 2nd ed. Used by permission of the author.

LABORATORY RESULTS SPECIFIC FOR DISEASES

Disease	Decreased Levels	Increased Levels
Cirrhosis	WBC Hemoglobin Hematocrit Albumin Sodium Potassium Chloride Magnesium Cholinesterase Vitamin A Vitamin B_{12} Vitamin C Vitamin K Folic acid Iron	Globulin Total bilirubin Alkaline phosphatase Transaminase LDH Anemia Neutropenia Thrombocytopenia Galactose intolerance Urine bilirubin Stool urobilinogen Urine urobilinogen
Pancreatitis	Calcium	Serum amylase (in first 48 hours) Lipase WBC Glucose (up to 900 mg/100 ml) Hematocrit
DIC	Platelet count Fibrinogen	Protime PTT FSP or FDP

MICROSCOPIC EXAMINATION OF URINE

Microscopic Element	Normal	Abnormal	Possible Implications
Red blood cells Adult Child	1 to 3 per high-power field Rare RBCs	More than 3 per HPF More than 1 per HPF	Inflammation or tumor of the urinary tract Subacute bacterial endocarditis Catheterization trauma Drugs tylenol, amphotericin B, ASA, coumarin, indomethacin, thiazides, sulfonamides Urinary calculi Papillary necrosis Sickle-cell disease Acute tubular necrosis Menstruation
White blood cells Adult Child	0 to 4 per HPF 0 to 4 per HPF	More than 4 per HPF	Infection—renal or urinary tract Renal disease Febrile illness Drugs: ampicillin, allopurinal, karamycin, methicillin, levodopa

MICROSCOPIC EXAMINATION OF URINE

Microscopic Element	Normal	Abnormal	Possible Implications
Squamous epithelial cells Adult Child	 Few Few	 Many Many	Contaminated specimen Tubular degeneration Presence of vaginal discharge Drugs: ASA, acetaminophen calcitonin, cortisone
Hyaline casts Adult Child	 Few Rare	 Many Few	Renal disease after diuretic therapy Dehydration Inflammation
Granular casts	None	Present	Totally carbohyrate diet Damage to urinary tract (if many present) Lead poisoning
White blood cell casts	None	Present	Lupus erythematosus Inflammation Pyelonephritis— (acute or chronic)

MICROSCOPIC EXAMINATION OF URINE

Microscopic Element	Normal	Abnormal	Possible Implications
Red blood cell casts	None	Present	Glomerulonephritis Vasculitis Periarteritis nodosa Tubular necrosis
Crystals Adult Child	 Few Few	Urate Many (oxalate) Many	Indicative of gout Possible passage of calculus (with ureteral colic hx) Drugs: (acetazolamide, vitamin C, nitrofurantoin, theophylline, thiazides) Liver disease
Bacteria Adult Child	 Few None	More than 100,000 per ml	Old specimen Infection
Yeast Adult Child	 Few None	 Many Present	Genitourinary infection Contaminated specimen

LABORATORY FINDINGS SUGGESTIVE OF MEDICAL DISORDERS

Test	Abnormally high levels	Abnormally low levels
ELECTROLYTES		
Calcium	Acidosis Acute renal failure Bone metastases Carcinoma Hypervitaminosis D Adrenal hypofunction Hyperparathyroidism Hyperthyroidism	Hypoparathyroidism Renal insufficiency Renal tubular acidosis Cushing's syndrome Acute pancreatitis Ulcerative colitis
Chloride	Diabetes insipidus Hyperparathyroidism Renal tubular acidosis	Burns Primary hyperaldosteronism Adrenal hypofunction CHF
Magnesium	Adrenal hypofunction Early stage diabetic acidosis Hypothyroidism Renal failure	Hyperparathyroidism Hyperthyroidism Primary hyperaldosteronism Malabsorption Malnutrition

LABORATORY FINDINGS SUGGESTIVE OF MEDICAL DISORDERS

Test	Abnormally high levels	Abnormally low levels
Phosphate	Addison's disease Acromegaly Hypoparathyroidism Renal insufficiency Bone metastases Diabetic acidosis	Hyperparathyroidism Diabetes Renal tubular disorders
Potassium	Hypoaldosteronism Adrenal hypofunction Circulatory failure Diabetes mellitus Renal insufficiency Respiratory acidosis Shock Massive tranfusions Hyperparathyroidism Heatstroke	Cushing's syndrome Primary hyper-aldosteronism Alkalosis Hepatic coma Diarrhea Vomiting Congestive heart failure Paralytic ileus Diuresis Excessive licorice ingestion

LABORATORY FINDINGS SUGGESTIVE OF MEDICAL DISORDERS

Test	Abnormally high levels	Abnormally low levels
Sodium	Acute renal failure CNS disorders Salicylate toxicity Osmotic diuresis Cushing's syndrome Diabetes insipidus Hyperosmolar hyperglycemic nonketotic coma (HHNC) Primary hyperaldosteronism	Adrenal hypofunction Chronic primary adrenocortical insufficiency Cirrhosis with ascites Guillain-Barré syndrome Burns SIADH Diabetic ketoacidosis
BLOOD CHEMISTRY		
Albumin	Diabetic acidosis Hypothyroidism	Malabsorption Burns Hyperthyroidism Hypocalcemia Chronic liver disease Carcinoma

LABORATORY FINDINGS SUGGESTIVE OF MEDICAL DISORDERS

Test	Abnormally high levels	Abnormally low levels
Alkaline phosphatase	Chronic renal failure Acromegaly Hyperparathyroidism Hyperthyroidism Liver disease Biliary obstruction Bone metastases Mononucleosis Pancreatitis Ulcerative colitis	Hypothyroidism Pernicious anemia Malnutrition Hypophosphatemia Milk-Alkali syndrome Celiac disease
Bicarbonate	Cushing's syndrome	Adrenal hypofunction
Blood urea nitrogen	Adrenal hypofunction Uncontrolled diabetes mellitus GI bleeding Renal insufficiency Shock Sepsis Burns	Acromegaly Liver failure Nephrotic sydrome Overhydration
Cholesterol	Hypothyroidism Diabetes mellitus Pregnancy Hepatic disease Pancreatitis	Hyperthyroidism Sepsis Acute infections Anemias

LABORATORY FINDINGS SUGGESTIVE OF MEDICAL DISORDERS

Test	Abnormally high levels	Abnormally low levels
Creatinine	Uncontrolled diabetes mellitus Adrenal hypofunction Renal insufficiency Pre-renal azotemia	
Glucose	Acromegaly Cushing's syndrome Diabetes mellitus Hyperpituitarism Pheochromocytoma Hyperthyroidism Acute pancreatitis Sepsis Tumors Anoxia Burns Seizures Stress MI Shock Hyperglycemia Hyperosmolar non-ketotic coma (HHNC)	Adrenal hypofunction Hypopituitarism Hypothyroidism Insulinoma Bacterial sepsis Malnutrition/ malabsorption G-6-PD deficiency Cirrhosis Reye's syndrome

LABORATORY FINDINGS SUGGESTIVE OF MEDICAL DISORDERS

Test	Abnormally high levels	Abnormally low levels
Lactic dehydrogenase (LDH)	Hypothyroidism Severe diabetic acidosis Carcinoma Pancreatitis Cirrhosis Hepatitis Hemolytic anemia Seizures Leukemia Myocardial infarction Drugs such as: ASA, mithramycin procainamide	

LABORATORY FINDINGS SUGGESTIVE OF MEDICAL DISORDERS

Test	Abnormally high levels	Abnormally low levels
Serum glutamic-oxaloascetic transaminase (SGOT)	Hypothyroidism Diabetic acidosis Hemolytic anemia Myocardial infarction Cirrhosis Pericarditis Hepatitis Pancreatitis Severe burns Shock Primary muscle disease Eclampsia Drugs such as: warfarin, digoxin, contraceptives opiates, salicylates	Pregnancy Beriberi
Total Protein	Diabetic acidosis Hypothyroidism Leukemia Multiple myeloma Shock Tuberculosis	Chronic uncontrolled diabetes mellitus Hyperthyroidism Pancreatitis Cirrhosis Hemorrhage Ulcerative colitis Malnutrition Malabsorption Cushing's syndrome Thyrotoxicosis Nephrotic syndrome

LABORATORY FINDINGS SUGGESTIVE OF MEDICAL DISORDERS

Test	Abnormally high levels	Abnormally low levels
HEMATOLOGY		
Hematocrit	Polycythemia Adrenal hypofunction Cushing's syndrome Dehydration Diabetic acidosis Pheochromocytoma Chronic obstructive lung disease	Hemorrhage Anemia Overhydration DIC Renal failure
Hemoglobin	Chronic obstructive lung disease Polycythemia Cushing's syndrome Pheochromocytoma Dehydration	Hemorrhage Anemias DIC Renal failure Ectopic ACH syndrome Hypopituitarism Hypothyroidism
Red blood cells	Pituitary tumors Polycythemia Chronic hypoxia	Adrenal hypofunction Hemolysis Aplastic anemia Hemorrhage Renal failure DIC

COLLOID ONCOTIC PRESSURE (COP)

COP = (1.4 × globulin) + (5.5 × albumin)

If PCWP − COP is less than 8, the probability is high for non-cardiogenic pulmonary edema.

SERUM OSMOLALITY

$$\text{Serum Osmolality} = (2 \times \text{Na}) + \frac{\text{BUN}}{3} + \frac{\text{GLUCOSE}}{18}$$

Normal: 285

With osmolality of 360 or above, confusion, seizures, and coma occur.

Sodium less than or equal to 115 equals a medical emergency. Patient needs 3% saline replacement.

PLATELETS

Spontaneous bleeding can occur with platelets less than 20,000.

Drugs that can alter platelet action include: ethanol, aspirin, quinidine, indocin, persantine, butazolidine, anturane, and atromid.

Treatment—IV platelets should increase platelet count by 10-15,000. If it does not, either a hypersplenic condition or antibody problem exists in which something is killing the platelets.

46 Laboratory Values

ROUTINE URINALYSIS

TEST	ADULT NORM	CHILD NORM	INCREASED VALUE MAY MEAN	DECREASED VALUE MAY MEAN
Color	Straw	Straw	**Dark:** Concentrated urine **Yellow-green:** Obstructive jaundice **Dark brown or black:** Increased dose of levodopa; intestinal obstruction; Addison's disease **Red:** Menstrual contamination; foods (beets, rhubarb); urinary tract bleeding; food dyes **Bright yellow:** Vitamin B_2; carotene **Blue-green:** Methylene blue dye; *Pseudomonas* infection	Diluted urine

ROUTINE URINALYSIS

TEST	ADULT NORM	CHILD NORM	INCREASED VALUE MAY MEAN	DECREASED VALUE MAY MEAN
Clarity	Clear	Clear	**Cloudy, white:** Pyuria; spermatazoa; fecal contamination; mucous strands; tissue **Opalescent:** Bacteria **Milky:** Degenerative tubular disease; crush injuries; lymphatic obstruction **Smoky:** Red blood cells **Pink, cloudy:** Uric acid	
Specific gravity	1.005-1.030	1.001-1.020	Dehydration; X-ray dye; IV albumin; trauma; stress; increased ADH; old specimen	Diabetes insipidus; renal tubular damage; cold urine
pH	4.5-8	5.0-7.0	Old specimen; metabolic alkalosis; respiratory alkalosis; renal tubular acidosis, renal tubular acidosis; increased gastric acid; vegetarianism; infection; immobilization; drugs	Sleep; high protein diet; respiratory acidosis; diabetes mellitus; diarrhea; fever; drugs

ROUTINE URINALYSIS

TEST	ADULT NORM	CHILD NORM	INCREASED VALUE MAY MEAN	DECREASED VALUE MAY MEAN
Protein	Negative	Negative	Mushroom poisoning; reaction to poison oak or ivy; electroshock therapy; dehydration; strenuous exercise; hemorrhage; sodium depletion; fever; stress; renal disease; glomerulonephritis; nephrotoxicity; pyelonephritis; renal tubular acidosis; urinary tract infection	Dilute urine; very alkaline urine
Glucose	Negative	Negative	**With concurrent hyperglycemia:** Diabetes mellitus; pituitary disorders; adrenal disorders; liver disease; pancreatic disease; hyperthyroidism; pheochromocytoma; burns; shock; fractures; infection; MI; increased carbohydrate diet; pregnancy **Without concurrent hyperglycemia:** Renal tubular dysfunction; poisoning; pregnancy; Fanconi's syndrome	

ROUTINE URINALYSIS

TEST	ADULT NORM	CHILD NORM	INCREASED VALUE MAY MEAN	DECREASED VALUE MAY MEAN
Keytones	Negative	Negative	Uncontrolled diabetes mellitus; nausea/vomiting/diarrhea; starvation; hyperthyroidism; ketogenic diet; hypoglycemia	
Occult blood	Negative	Negative	Drugs; strenuous exercise; post transfusions; hemolytic anemias; thrombotic thrombocytopenia purpura; malaria; burns; lupus erythematosus; viral infections; uremic syndrome	

50 Laboratory Values

EFFECTS OF DRUGS ON ROUTINE URINALYSIS

TEST	INCREASED TEST VALUES	DECREASED TEST VALUES
Color (red or pink)	Food dyes Levodopa Phenolphthalein Rifampin Sulfobromophthalein	Ethanol
Color (orange, orange-red, yellow-orange)	Cascara sagrada Chlorzoxazone Indandione Anticoagulants Phenazopyridine HCl Sulfasalazine	
Color (yellow)	Fluorescein injections Vitamin B_2 Quinacrine	
Color (green-blue)	Magnesium salicylate Indomethacin Methylene blue Triamterene	
Color (brown, brown-red, dark)	Auralgan otic solution Cascara sagrada Chloroquine Furazolidone Iron preparations Mentronidazole Nitrofurantoin Bacitracin Co-trimoxazole	

EFFECTS OF DRUGS ON ROUTINE URINALYSIS

TEST	INCREASED TEST VALUES	DECREASED TEST VALUES
Cloudy	Carbonates Phosphates X-ray contrast media	
Specific Gravity	Albumin Dextran Glucose X-ray contrast media	Methoxyflurane
pH	Acetazolamide Amphotericin B Epinephrine Niacinamide Parathyroid hormone Triamterene	Ascorbic acid ACTH Diazoxide Glucose Methenamine Metolazone Niacin

EFFECTS OF DRUGS ON ROUTINE URINALYSIS

TEST	INCREASED TEST VALUES	DECREASED TEST VALUES
Protein	Acetaminophen Amphotericin B Ampicillin Aspirin Bacitracin Chlorpropamide Codeine Corticosteroids Edetate Chlorhexidine gluconate Furosemide Gentamicin Gold Griseofulvin Heroin Kanamycin Methicillin Neomycin Probenecid Acetazolamide X-ray contrast media Bicarbonates	

EFFECTS OF DRUGS ON ROUTINE URINALYSIS

TEST	INCREASED TEST VALUES	DECREASED TEST VALUES
Glucose	Aspirin Carbamazepine Chlorpromazine Chlorthalidone Corticosteroids Dextrothyroxine sodium Lithium Phenothiazines Thiazides	Ampicillin Ascorbic acid Bisacodyl Chloral hydrate Diazepam Digoxin Epinephrine Ferrous sulfate Furosemide Levodopa Phenobarbital Prednisone Secobarbital Some vitamin preparations
Ketones	Aspirin Ethanol Ether High doses of insulin Ioniazid High doses of isopropanol Niacin	
Occult blood	Hypochlorites	

CEREBROSPINAL FLUID LAB VALUES

Condition	Pressure	Appearance	Cell Makeup	Protein	Glucose	Chloride
Normal Adult	60-80 mm H2O	Clear	0-5 Lymphs	15-45 mg/dl	40-80 mg/dl 2.75-4.40 mmol/L	700-750 mg/dl 120-130 mEq/L 120-130 mmol/L (SI)
Normal Child	50-100 mm H2O	Clear	0-8 lymphs mm^3	15-48 mg/dl	35-75 mg/dl	122-128 mEq/L
Intracranial abscess	Elevated	Clear but may be discolored	Normal to elevated	Normal to increased	Normal to decreased	Normal
Cerebral infarct	Elevated	Clear	Increased	Increased	Normal	Normal
Subarachnoid hemorrhage	Normal to extreme elevation	Pink to red	Increased in red and white cells	Increased	Normal to decreased	Normal

CEREBROSPINAL FLUID LAB VALUES

Condition	Pressure	Appearance	Cell Makeup	Protein	Glucose	Chloride
Bacterial meningitis	Moderate to extreme elevation	Clear to purulent	Increase in white cells usually 10-50 k	Increased	Decreased	Decreased
Tumor	Elevated	Clear	Elevated	Increased	Increased with hypothalamic tumor	

56 Laboratory Values

MEDICATIONS AND MEDICATION CHARTS

58 *Medications and Medication Charts*

TABLE OF CONTENTS

Commonly-used Medications	59
Apresoline Drip Chart	212
Tridil Table	213
Starting Rates for Vasoactive Drugs	214
Method for Rapid Calculation of IV Drips	215
Inocor Chart	218
Nipride Chart	219
Dobutamine Chart	224
Dopamine Chart	226
Children's Dopamine Chart	229
Children's Dobutrex Chart	231
Cardiovascular Drugs	232

COMMONLY-USED MEDICATIONS

Note: While drugs are mixed in mg, dosing of some drugs is done in µg/kg/min..

✤ acebutolol

Trade: Monitan, Sectral

Classification:

Cardioselective β–blocker with antiarrhythmic effects

Action:

- Competitively blocks stimulation of β-adrenergic receptor
- Produces chronotropic, inotropic activity
- Slows conduction of AV node
- Decreases heart rate, B/P and cardiac output

Decreases myocardial oxygen consumption

- Decreases renin-aldosterone-angiotensin system at high doses
- Inhibits β–2 receptors in the bronchial system at high doses

Clinical Applications:

Useful in treating mild to moderate hypertension, sinus tachycardia, persistent atrial extrasystoles, tachydysrhythmias, and for prophylaxis of angina.

Dose:

Hypertension

Adult: 400 mg PO qd or in 2 divided doses, maximum 1200 mg/day

Dysrhythmias

Adult: 200 mg PO bid, may increase gradually, usual dosage 600-1200 mg daily.

Side Effects:

CNS: Catatonia, depression, dizziness, fatigue, hallucinations, insomnia, mental changes

CV: Bradycardia, CHF, second and third degree heart block, hypotension

GI: Diarrhea, ischemic colitis, nausea, vomiting, mesenteric arterial thrombosis

GU: Impotence

RESP: Bronchospasm, dyspnea

INTEG: Alopecia, fever, cold extremities, rash

HEMA: Agranulocytosis, purpura, thrombocytopenia

EENT: Dry eyes, sore throat

Nursing Considerations:

Assess VS; notify MD for pulse < 60/min or significant changes in B/P. Baseline liver and renal function lab prior to med administration. Assess I&O; monitor edema to extremities; weigh daily. Monitor for increased levels in lab studies. Do not discontinue drug abruptly, as this may cause angina. Taper over two weeks. Maintain fluid balance; monitor turgor, mucous membranes, hydration. Do not use over-the-counter cough, cold or allergy meds without MD approval.

Precautions:

Increased hypoglycemia may occur with concurrent use of insulin. Use with caution in pregnancy (B), lactation, diabetes, COPD, asthma, valvular heart disease, renal or thyroid disease. Catecholamine-depleting drugs may have additive effects.

Contraindications:

Cardiogenic shock, advanced AV block, bradycardia, cardiac failure and with concurrent general anesthesia.

✤ acyclovir sodium

Trade: Zovirax

Classification:

Antiviral

Action:

- Interferes with DNA synthesis
- Inhibits replication

Clinical Application:

Used in the treatment of genital herpes, herpes simplex, varicella-zoster virus, Epstein-Barr virus, cytomegalovirus, and herpes simplex encephalitis.

Dose:

Herpes Simplex

Adult: 5 mg/kg IV over 1 hour q8h for 5 days

Child >12 yrs: 250 mg/m^2 over 1 hour q8h for 5 days

Genital Herpes

Adult: 200 mg PO q4h for 5 days; may be given for up to 6 months in chronic cases

Herpes Simplex Encephalitis

Child > 6 mo. but < 1 yr: 500 mg/m^2 IV over 1 hr q8h for 10 days

Side Effects:

CNS: Chills, coma, confusion, convulsions, hallucinations, headache, lightheadedness, psychosis

CV: Cardiac tamponade, chest pain, edema, hypotension

GI: Anorexia, abdominal pain, increased liver function tests, nausea

GU: Anuria, dysuria, hematuria, renal failure, increased BUN and creatinine, increased urinary sediment

RESP: Pulmonary edema

INTEG: Diaphoresis, fever, ischemia to fingers and toes, phlebitis, rash

HEMA: Anemia, hypokalemia, leukopenia, neutropenia, thrombocytopenia

Nursing Considerations:

Monitor I&O. Notify MD for decrease in urine output < 30 cc/hr, hematuria, or increased sedimentation. Maintain fluid status; if warranted, increase fluids to 3 L/day. Obtain C&S prior to institution of therapy and after antibiotic therapy.

Assess liver function studies, renal function studies, signs/symptoms of infection, blood studies, bleeding times for abnormalities. Use only solutions without preservatives to reconstitute medication.

Precautions:

Use with caution in renal or hepatic disease, electrolyte imbalance, dehydration, lactation and pregnancy (C).

Contraindications:

Hypersensitivity to drug

✤ adenosine

Trade: Adenocard

Classification:

Antidysrhythmic

Action:

- Decreases conduction through AV node
- Can interrupt reentry pathways through the AV node
- May produce a transient AV block or asystole

Clinical Applications:

Used for the treatment to convert paroxysmal supraventricular tachycardias to sinus rhythm.

Dose:

Adult: 6 mg IV bolus, rapidly; if conversion to normal sinus rhythm does not occur within 1-2 min, give 12 mg by rapid IV bolus, may repeat 12 mg dose again

Side Effects:

CNS: Apprehension, dizziness, headache, lightheadedness, numbness, arm tingling

CV: Asystole, chest pain or pressure, heart block, hypotension, palpitations, atrial tachydysrhythmias

GI: Nausea, throat tightness

GU: Groin pressure

EENT: Blurred vision, metallic taste

INTEG: Facial flushing, sweating

Nursing Considerations:

Continuous cardiac monitoring must be used. Monitor VS for fluctuations. Flush IV line with solution rapidly after IV bolus

Precautions:

Use with caution in pregnancy (C), lactation, children, asthma, or elderly. Adenosine effects are potentiated with use of dipyridamole and antagonized by methylxanthines (caffeine, theophylline).

Contraindications:

Advanced heart block, sick sinus syndrome, atrial flutter or fibrillation, or ventricular ectopy

---

✣ alteplase

Trade: Activase

Classification:

Antithrombotic

- Converts plasminogen in thrombus to plasmin
- Binds to fibrin
- Causes local fibrinolysis and limited systemic proteolysis

Clinical Application:

Used for the treatment of lysis of thrombi in myocardial infarction and for lysis of acute pulmonary emboli

Dose:

Adult: 6-10 mg IV bolus over 1-2 minutes, then 60 mg IV over the first hour, 20 mg/hr IV over the second and third hours

Adult weighing < 65 kg: 1.25 mg/kg IV over 3 hours.

To mix, reconstitute with provided diluent, add 20 cc sterile water for injection to 20 mg vial or 50 cc to 50 mg vial. Slowly rotate —DO NOT SHAKE.

Side Effects:

CNS: Intracranial bleeding

CV: Accelerated idioventricular rhythm, sinus bradycardia, dysrhythmias, hypotension, ventricular tachycardia

GI: Bleeding, nausea, vomiting

GU: Hematuria

EENT: Epistaxis, oral bleeding

INTEG: Ecchymoses, fever, rash, urticaria

RESP: Laryngeal edema, hemoptysis

Nursing Considerations:

Continuous cardiac monitoring for dysrhythmias and reperfusion dysrhythmias. Monitor VS, neurological status, peripheral pulses, and notify MD for significant changes. Assess heart and lung sounds. Assess for bleeding from all areas, guaiac all body fluids and stools. No ABGs unless absolutely mandatory, and then apply pressure for at least 30 minutes. No needlesticks unless necessary and venipunctures should be done with needle gauge no larger than 22. Pressure dressings must be applied to all puncture sites.

Monitor lab studies before and after therapy, including cardiac enzymes, CBC, and electrolytes. Anticipate use of heparin after alteplase discontinued or when ACT or APTT less than 2 times control value. Flush line/container with NS after administration. Do not use solution with preservatives.

Precautions:

Use with caution in pregnancy (C), lactation, recent major surgery, cerebrovascular disease, mitral stenosis, pericarditis, subacute bacterial endocarditis, hepatic or renal disease, septic thrombophlebitis, or concurrent oral anticoagulant use.

Contraindications:

Hypersensitivity, active bleeding, recent CVA, uncontrolled hypertension, intracranial or intraspinal surgery, trauma, children, aneurysm, or AV malformation.

✣ amphotericin B

Trade: Amphotericin B, Fungizone IV

Classification:

Antifungal antibiotic

Action:

- Binds to steroids on cell membranes
- Changes permeability of cell membranes

Clinical Application:

Used for severe and life-threatening fungal infections, such as aspergillosis, blastomycosis, systemic candidiasis, coccidioidomycosis histoplasmosis, meningitis, sporotrichosis, and mucocutaneous leishmaniasis.

Dose:

Test dose

1 mg in 20 cc D$_5$W IV over 20-30 minutes while monitoring VS

Infection

Adult: 1 mg in 250 cc D$_5$W IV over 2-4 hours, or 0.25 mg/kg IV daily over 6 hrs; may increase to 1 mg/kg/day up to a maximum of 1.5 mg/kg/day; [To mix solution, mix 5 mg of drug with 10 cc sterile water without preservatives, then further dilute in 250-500 cc D$_5$W]

Child: Same as adult

Side Effects:

CNS: Chills, convulsions, dizziness, fever, headache, paresthesia, peripheral nerve pain, peripheral neuropathy

CV: Arrest, cardiac failure, dysrhythmias, hypotension, hypertension

GI: Anorexia, cramps, diarrhea, hemorrhagic gastroenteritis, liver failure, nausea, vomiting

GU: Azotemia, anuria, hyposthenuria, hypokalemia, nephrocalcinosis, oliguria, renal impairment, renal tubular acidosis

RESP: Bronchospasms, dyspnea, pneumonitis, pulmonary edema, tachypnea, wheezing

MS: Arthralgia, myalgia, weakness, weight loss

EENT: Blurred vision, deafness, diplopia, tinnitus

INTEG: Burning or pain at site, dermatitis, extravasation, flushing, pruritus, necrosis, skin rash, thrombophlebitis

HEMA: Agranulocytosis, anemia, eosinophilia, hypokalemia, hyponatremia, hypomagnesemia, leukopenia, thrombocytopenia

Nursing Considerations:

Monitor EKG for flattening of T waves, ST depression, widening of QRS, and notify MD of abnormalities. Monitor VS, including temperature q15-30 minutes for the first dose; notify MD for changes in heart rate or B/P. Do not use normal saline or solutions with preservatives to reconstitute medication. Use an in-line filter with pore diameter ≤ 1.0 microns. Protect solution from the light; wrap container with aluminum foil. Monitor I&O; notify MD for urine output < 30cc/hr. Weigh patient daily and notify MD for significant changes. Monitor lab for CBC, renal studies, calcium and magnesium level abnormalities. Assess for rash or ototoxicity. Side effects can be decreased with use of aspirin, acetaminophen, antihistamines and/or antiemetics.

Precautions:

Use with caution in decreased renal function, pregnancy (B), concurrent use of antineoplastics, steroids, ACTH, digoxin, imidazoles, aminoglycosides, skeletal muscle relaxants and leukocyte transfusions.

Contraindications:

Hypersensitivity to drug or severe bone marrow depression.

✣ amrinone lactate

Trade: Inocor

Classification:

Cardiac inotropic agent

Action:

- Rapid-acting positive inotropic with vasodilator properties
- Inhibits phosphodiesterase activity
- Enhances myocardial contractility
- Increases cardiac output and stroke volume
- Reduces right and left ventricular filling pressures by direct relaxation on vascular smooth muscle
- Decreases pulmonary capillary wedge pressure (PCWP), systemic vascular resistance (SVR), total peripheral resistance (TPR), and peripheral vascular resistance (PVR)
- Decreases preload and afterload

Clinical Applications:

Used for the short-term management of congestive heart failure in patients not responding to other medications; may be used with digitalis

Dose:

Adult: 0.75 mg/kg IV bolus loading dose over 2-3 minutes, followed by infusion with drip (500 mg/100 cc NS or 0.45% NS) at 2-10 µg/kg/min, and titrated for optimum hemodynamics

A second bolus dose can be given after 30 min, if necessary. Maximum recommended dose: 10 mg/kg/day with rare instances of up to 18 mg/kg/day for short duration

Side Effects:

CV: Chest pain, dysrhythmias, headache, hypotension, pericarditis

GI: Abdominal pain, anorexia, ascites, hepatotoxicity, hiccoughs, jaundice, nausea, vomiting

RESP: Hypoxemia, pleuritis, pulmonary denseness

HEMA: Thrombocytopenia

INTEG: Allergic reactions, fever

Nursing Considerations:

Continuous cardiac monitoring should be used. Notify MD of dysrhythmias; assess B/P and pulse q5-15 min during active titration. Notify MD, and stop infusion for decrease of B/P 30 mm Hg or more. Strict I&O; weigh patient daily. Assess for edema, hydration status.

Lab: Electrolytes, renal studies, platelet count as ordered. (If platelets decrease below 150,000/mm^3, Inocor usually discontinued) ALT, AST, bilirubin q1-2 days. Drug should not be mixed with dextrose solutions, or with any other medication. Lasix will cause a precipitate to form.

Precautions:

Use with caution in pregnancy (C), renal, or hepatic disease, atrial flutter/fibrillation, elderly, children, lactation, uncorrected hypokalemia, or dehydration

Contraindications:

Hypersensitivity to this drug or bisulfites, severe valvular disease, or acute MI

✢ atenolol

Trade: Atenolol, Tenormin

Classification:

Cardioselective β-blocker

Action:

- Blocks stimulation of the β-receptors in vascular smooth muscle
- Decreases the rate of SA node discharge and increases recovery time
- Slows conduction of the AV node
- Decreases the heart rate, B/P and cardiac output
- Decreases myocardial oxygen consumption
- Decreases the renin-aldosterone-angiotensin system at high doses
- Inhibits bronchial system β–receptors at high doses

Clinical Applications:
Useful in treating mild to moderate hypertension, for prophylaxis in anginal pain, and in treatment of known or suspected MI.

Dose:
Adult: 5 mg IV given over 5 min, or diluted in 25-50 cc of D5W, 0.45% NS, or 0.9% NS and given as an intermittent infusion; a second dose may be repeated in 10 min if the patient tolerates the first dose, and then a PO dose is started 10 min after the last IV dose

50 mg PO qd; increase dose q1-2 weeks to 100 mg qd; may increase up to 200 mg PO qd for angina

Side Effects:

CNS: Catatonia, depression, dizziness, fatigue, hallucinations, insomnia, memory loss, mental changes

CV: Bradycardia, cold extremities, CHF, profound hypotension, second and third degree heart blocks

GI: Diarrhea, ischemic colitis, nausea, mesenteric arterial thrombosis, vomiting

GU: Impotence, renal failure

RESP: Bronchospasm, dyspnea, wheezing

EENT: Dry eyes, sore throat

HEMA: Agranulocytosis, purpura, thrombocytopenia

INTEG: Alopecia, fever, rash

Nursing Considerations:

Assess VS; notify MD of significant changes in B/P or pulse. Baseline renal and liver function studies prior to administration of drug. Assess I&O; monitor edema to lower extremities, turgor, mucous membranes. Maintain fluid balance; weigh daily. Do not use over-the-counter cough, cold or allergy medications without MD approval. Do not discontinue drug abruptly; taper over two weeks.

Precautions:

Use with caution in pregnancy (C), lactation, diabetes, major surgery, COPD, asthma, and renal or thyroid disease.

Contraindications:

Cardiogenic shock, advanced heart blocks, bradycardia, and cardiac failure; incompatible with any other drug or solution in syringe.

✤ atropine

Trade: Atropine

Classification:

Anticholinergic-parasympatholytic

Action:

- Parasympatholytic drug that induces sinus node automaticity
- Improves AV conduction

- May restore normal AV nodal conduction and initiate electrical activity during asystole
- Increases SA node discharge
- Blocks vagal impulse to SA node, atria, and AV node, and increases cardiac output and heart rate

Clinical Applications:

Used in symptomatic bradycardias, sinus arrest and block, asystole, bradydysrhythmias. Administered as a treatment for anticholinesterase insecticide poisoning, as an agent to decrease secretions prior to surgery, and as a bronchodilator.

Dose:

Bradycardias

Adult: 0.5-1 mg IV bolus over 1 min; may repeat as needed up to a maximum of 0.04 mg/kg/24 hrs

Child: 0.01-0.03 mg/kg IV bolus over 1 min; may repeat as needed up to a maximum of 0.4 mg, or 0.3 mg/m^2

Pre-op

Adult: 0.4-0.5 mg IV, IM, SQ prior to anesthesia

Child: 0.1-0.3 mg SQ 30 min prior to surgery

Poisoning

Adult: 2 mg IM, IV q1h until symptoms abate, may need up to 6 mg/hr.

Child: Same as adult

Side Effects:

CNS: Anxiety, coma, confusion, dizziness, drowsiness, headache, insomnia, involuntary movements, psychosis

CV: Angina, rebound bradycardia, hypotension, hypertension, tachycardia, ventricular ectopy, ventricular fibrillation

GI: Anorexia, abdominal distention or pain, constipation, dry mouth, nausea, vomiting, paralytic ileus

GU: Dysuria, impotence, retention

INTEG: Contact dermatitis, dry skin, flushing, rash, urticaria

EENT: Blurred vision, eye pain, glaucoma, pupil dilation, photophobia

Nursing Considerations:

Cardiac monitoring should be used for bradydysrhythmia problems. Assess for decreased urinary output or retention, constipation, respiratory changes, such as dyspnea, cyanosis, wheezing or distended neck veins.

Precautions:

Use with caution in myocardial ischemia or infarction, pregnancy (C), lactation, CHF, children younger than 6 years, COPD, renal or hepatic disease, hypertension, and hyperthyroidism

Contraindications:

Hypersensitivity to belladonna alkaloids, GI obstruction, myasthenia gravis, angle-closure glaucoma, asthma, thyrotoxicosis, ulcerative colitis, prostatic hypertrophy, or tachydysrhythmias

✤ bretylium tosylate

Trade: Bretylate, Bretylium Tosylate, Bretylol

Classification:

Antidysrhythmic (Class III)

Action:

- Produces antiarrhythmic effects
- Releases norepinephrine from the adrenergic nerve endings in direct relation to its concentration at the adrenergic terminal
- Increases heart rate transiently
- Increases cardiac output
- Potentiates the action of catecholamines
- Prolongs the action potential duration and elevates ventricular fibrillation threshold

Clinical Applications:

Used for the treatment of ventricular fibrillation or life-threatening ventricular tachycardia, refractory to other therapy.

Dose:

Adult: 5 mg/kg IV bolus, over 15-30 seconds *if patient is unconscious*; over 1-2 min if patient is conscious. If ventricular fibrillation persists, a dose of 10 mg/kg is given and repeated at 15 to 30 minute intervals for maximum of 30 mg/kg; follow with drip (2 gm/500 cc of D_5W or 0.9% NS) at 1-4 mg/min)

Side Effects:

CNS: Anxiety, confusion, dizziness, syncope

CV: Angina, bradycardia, hypotension, transient hypertension, PVCs, substernal pressure

GI: Diarrhea, hiccups, immediate nausea, vomiting

GU: Renal dysfunction

RESP: Respiratory depression, shortness of breath

INTEG: Flushing, rash

Nursing Considerations:

Continuous cardiac monitoring must be observed. Assess B/P and pulse q5-15 min initially to monitor drug response and to observe for rebound hypertension after 1-2 hours. Monitor I&O; weigh daily. Notify MD for urinary output < 30 cc/hr; patient should be kept supine until a tolerance to hypotension develops.

Precautions:

Give slowly in conscious patients to avoid vomiting. Use with caution in patients with renal disease, pregnancy (C).

Contraindications:

Digitoxin-induced arrhythmias, aortic stenosis, pulmonary hypertension and with children

✤ bumetanide

Trade: Bumex

Classification:

Loop diuretic

Action:
- Increases the excretion of sodium and chloride in the ascending loop of Henle

Clinical Applications:

Used in treating edema associated with CHF, pulmonary edema, ascites, and hypertension

Dose:

Adult: 0.5-2.0 mg PO qd; may repeat a second or third dose at 4-6 hour intervals, with maximum of 20 mg/day; IV/IM dose: 0.5-1.0 mg qd; may give a second or third dose at 2-4 hour intervals, with maximum of 20 mg/day

Side Effects:

CNS: Encephalopathy, headache

CV: Chest pain, circulatory collapse, EKG changes, hypotension

GI: Anorexia, abdominal pain, cramps, diarrhea, dry mouth, jaundice, nausea, acute pancreatitis, vomiting

GU: Glycosuria, polyuria, renal failure

EENT: Blurred vision, ear pain, hearing loss, tinnitus

INTEG: Photosensitivity, pruritus, purpura, rash, sweating

MS: Arthritis, muscular cramps, stiffness

HEMA: Agranulocytosis, neutropenia, thrombocytopenia

ENDO: Hyperglycemia, hyperuricemia, hypomagnesemia, hypocalcemia, hyponatremia

Nursing Considerations:

Assess I&O; weigh daily. Maintain fluid balance. If warranted, increase fluid intake to 2-3 L/day. Potassium replacement should occur for < 3.0 mg/dl level. Assess VS; observe for dyspnea with exertion and postural hypotension. Assess hearing for changes. Assess edema; monitor hydration with skin turgor and mucous membranes. Monitor serum electrolytes, renal function studies for increased uric acid levels. Administer in the morning to avoid nocturia.

Precautions:

Use with caution in dehydration, ascites, pregnancy (C), and severe renal or hepatic disease. Concurrent use with antihypertensives may cause an increased effect. Concurrent use with antidiabetics may cause a decreased effect.

Contraindications:

Anuria, hepatic coma, hypovolemia, or history of gout.

✣ calcium chloride

Trade: Calcium Chloride

Classification:

Electrolyte replacement

Action:

- Replenishes calcium
- Regulates excitation threshold of nerves and muscle
- Increases myocardial contractility
- Increases inotropic and toxic effects of digoxin
- Increases B/P

Clinical Applications:

Used for the treatment of hypermagnesemia, hyperkalemia, hypocalcemia, calcium-channel blocker toxicity, hyperphosphatemia, or Vitamin D deficiency.

Dose:

Adult: 500-1000 mg (5-10 cc of a 10% solution) IV over 5-10 minutes (no faster than 1 ml/min); may repeat as needed based on serum calcium levels, 200-800 mg injected into the ventricular cavity of the heart.

Child: 25 mg/kg IV over several min (rate should not exceed 0.5 ml/min)

Side Effects:

CNS: Coma, drowsiness, muscle weakness, sensation of tingling or heat waves, syncope

CV: Bradycardia, cardiac arrest, dysrhythmias, heart block, hypotension, shortened QT interval

GI: Constipation, nausea, vomiting

INTEG: Burning at IV site, extravasation, necrosis

GU: Polyuria, renal calculi

Nursing Considerations:

Continuous cardiac monitoring. Assess for shortened QT interval and T wave inversion. Calcium levels should be frequently obtained.

Precautions:

Use with caution in digitalized patient, respiratory failure, renal disease, children, and pregnancy (C). Do not give in same line as sodium bicarbonate.

Contraindications:

Ventricular fibrillation, hypercalcemia, digitalis toxicity and renal calculi

---

✣ captopril

Trade: Capoten

Classification:

Antihypertensive

Action:

- Inhibits conversion of angiotensin I to angiotensin II
- Dilates arterial and venous vessels
- Selectively suppresses the renin-aldosterone-angiotensin system
- Decreases B/P
- Increases renal blood flow

- Decreases peripheral vascular resistance, pulmonary capillary wedge pressure, systemic vascular resistance
- Increases cardiac output

Clinical Applications:

Used for the treatment of hypertension and for heart failure not responsive to other therapy.

Dose:

Adult: 12.5 mg PO bid or tid; may increase to 50 mg PO bid or tid at 1-2 week intervals; usual range is from 25-150 mg bid or tid, with maximum of 450 mg/day

Side Effects:

CNS: Dizziness, fatigue, headache, insomnia, paresthesia, seizures

CV: Angina, hypotension, palpitations, tachycardia

GI: Loss of taste, hepatitis, pancreatitis

GU: Dysuria, frequency, impotence, nephrotic syndrome, nocturia, oliguria, polyuria, proteinuria, acute reversible renal failure

RESP: Bronchospasm, cough, dyspnea

INTEG: Angioedema, fever, rash

HEMA: Anemia, neutropenia, thrombocytopenia, increased sedimentation rate

ENDO: Hyperkalemia

Nursing Considerations:

Assess VS, especially B/P. Monitor for worsening renal function on lab studies. Do not discontinue drug abruptly. Do not use over-the-counter cold or allergy products unless approved by physician. Assess for CHF, edema, dyspnea.

Precautions:

Use with caution in children, hypovolemia, leukemia, scleroderma, lupus erythematosus, blood dyscrasias, CHF, diabetes, renal or thyroid disease, COPD, asthma, or dialysis patients

Contraindications:

Pregnancy (C), lactation, and heart block

✤ cefamandole nafate

Trade: Mandol

Classification:

Antibiotic

Action

- Inhibits cell wall synthesis of bacterial organism
- Changes cell wall osmolality and causes cell death

Clinical Application:

Used in the treatment of skin infections, peritonitis, upper and lower respiratory tract, and urinary tract infections, septicemia, and for surgical prophylaxis. Used for gram positive bacteria (*S. pneumoniae, S. pyogenes, S. aureus*) and gram negative bacteria (*E. coli, P. mirabilis, Klebsiella,* and *H. influenzae*)

Dose:

Adult: 500-1000 mg IV q4-8h; mix in at least 10 cc of NS and given over 3-5 minutes, or can be further diluted in 50-100 cc and run over 15-30 min

Child > 1 mo: 50-100 mg/kg/day in divided doses q4-8h; do not exceed adult dose.

Side Effects:

CNS: Chills, dizziness, fever, headache, paresthesia, weakness

GI: Anorexia, increased AST, ALT, alkaline phosphatase, bilirubin, or LDH levels, bleeding, diarrhea, glossitis, nausea, pain, vomiting

GU: Increased BUN, candidiasis, nephrotoxicity, proteinuria, pruritus, renal failure, vaginitis

INTEG: Anaphylaxis, dermatitis, rash, urticaria

RESP: Dyspnea

HEMA: Agranulocytosis, anemia, hemolytic anemia, bleeding, eosinophilia, hypoprothrombinemia, leukopenia, lymphocytosis, pancytopenia, thrombocytopenia

Nursing Considerations:

Assess I&O; notify MD for urine output < 30 cc/hr. Monitor lab studies for worsening renal or hepatic function, or for blood dyscrasias. Assess bowel status and notify MD for severe diarrhea. Monitor IV site for infiltration and change as needed. Monitor for allergic reaction or bleeding.

Precautions:

Use with caution in pregnancy (B), lactation, or in renal disease, or patients with hypersensitivities to penicillin.

Contraindications:

Hypersensitivity to cephalosporins, infants younger than 1 month

---

✣ cefazolin sodium

Trade: Ancef, Cefazolin Sodium, Kefzol, Zolicef

Classification:
Antibiotic

Action

- Changes osmotic pressure in cell wall causing bacterial cell death
- Inhibits cell wall synthesis of bacterial organism

Clinical Application:

Used in the treatment of infections involving the skin, bones, joints, upper and lower respiratory tracts, urinary tract, genitals, and for endocarditis, septicemia, and surgical prophylaxis. Used for gram positive organisms (*S. aureus, S. pyogenes, and S. pneumoniae*) and gram negative organisms (*E. coli, P. mirabilis H. influenzae, and Klebsiella*).

Dose:

Adult: 1-1.5 g IV q6h; mix with at least 10 cc NS and give over 3-5 minutes; may be further diluted with 50-100 cc NS and run over 30 min

Child >1 mo.: 100 mg/kg/day in 3-4 divided doses

Less Severe Infections

Adult: 250-500 mg IV q8h

Child >1 mo.: 25-50 mg/kg/day in 3-4 divided doses

Side Effects:

CNS: Chills, dizziness, fever, headache, paresthesia, weakness

GI: Increased ALT, AST, alkaline phosphatase, bilirubin and LDH levels, abdominal pain, anorexia, bleeding, diarrhea, glossitis, nausea, vomiting

GU: Increased BUN, candidiasis, proteinuria, pruritus, nephrotoxicity, renal failure, vaginitis

INTEG: Anaphylaxis, dermatitis, rash urticaria

HEMA: Agranulocytosis, anemia, hemolytic anemia, eosinophilia, lymphocytosis, leukopenia, neutropenia, pancytopenia, thrombocytopenia

Nursing Considerations:

Assess I&O; notify MD for urine output < 30 cc/hr. Monitor lab studies for renal or hepatic function decrease, or blood dyscrasias. Monitor electrolytes for long-term therapy. Assess bowel status and notify MD for severe diarrhea. Monitor IV site for infiltration and change site as needed.

Precautions:

Use with caution in pregnancy (B), lactation, renal disease or hypersensitivity to penicillin

Contraindications:

Hypersensitivity to cephalosporins, infants younger than 1 month

---

✤ cefotaxime sodium

Trade: Claforan

Classification:

Antibiotic

Action:

- Inhibits cell wall synthesis
- Changes osmotic pressure in bacterial cell causing organism death

Clinical Application:

Used for the treatment of infections involving the skin, bones, lower respiratory tract, urinary tract, as well as gonococcal infections, bacteremia, septicemia, and meningitis. Used for gram positive organisms (*S. aureus, S. pyogenes, and S. pneumoniae*) and gram negative organisms (*E. coli, N. meningitidis, P. mirabilis, H. influenzae, N. gonnorrhoeae, Klebsiella, Citrobacter, Salmonella, Shigella, and Serratia*).

Dose:

Adult: 1 g IV q8-12h; mix with at least 10 cc D5W or NS and give over 3-5 minutes; may be further diluted in 50-100 cc of NS or D5W and given over 30 min.

Severe Infections

Adult: 2 g IV q4h; maximum of 12 g/day

Side Effects:

CNS: Chills, dizziness, fever, headache, paresthesia, weakness

GI: Increased ALT, AST, alkaline phosphatase, bilirubin and LDH levels, abdominal pain, anorexia, bleeding, diarrhea, glossitis, nausea, vomiting

GU: Increased BUN, candidiasis, nephrotoxicity, proteinuria, pruritus, renal failure, vaginitis

INTEG: Anaphylaxis, dermatitis, inflammation to site, pain, rash, urticaria

HEMA: Agranulocytosis, anemia, hemolytic anemia, eosinophilia, leukopenia, lymphocytosis, neutropenia, pancytopenia, thrombocytopenia

Nursing Considerations:

Assess I&O; notify MD for urine output < 30 cc/hr. Monitor lab studies for worsening renal or hepatic function or for blood dyscrasias. Monitor electrolytes if patient is on long-term therapy. Assess bowel status and notify MD for severe diarrhea. Assess IV site for infiltration and change site as needed.

Precautions:
Use with caution in pregnancy (B), lactation, renal disease, or hypersensitivity to penicillin

Contraindications:
Hypersensitivity to cephalosporins, infants younger than 1 month

---

✣ cefoxitin sodium

Trade: Mefoxin

Classification:
Antibiotic

Action:
- Inhibits cell wall synthesis of bacterial organisms
- Changes osmotic pressure in cell wall causing organism death

Clinical Application:
Used for the treatment of infections involving the skin, bones, urinary tract and lower respiratory tract, as well as gonococcal infections, septicemia, and peritonitis. Used for gram positive organisms (*S. aureus, S. pyogenes, S. pneumoniae*) and gram negative organism (*E. coli, H. influenzae, Proteus, Klebsiella, N. gonorrhoeae*).

Dose:
Adult: 1-2 g IV q6-8h; mix with at least 10 cc of NS or D_5W and give over 3-5 minutes; may be further diluted with 50-100 cc and run over 30 minutes

Severe Infections:

Adult: 2 g IV q4h

Side Effects:

CNS: Chills, dizziness, fever, headache, paresthesia, weakness

GI: Increased ALT, AST, alkaline phosphatase, bilirubin or LDH levels, abdominal pain, anorexia, bleeding, diarrhea, glossitis, nausea, vomiting

GU: Increased BUN, candidiasis, nephrotoxicity, proteinuria, pruritus, renal failure, vaginitis

INTEG: Anaphylaxis, dermatitis, rash, thrombophlebitis, urticaria

HEMA: Agranulocytosis, anemia, hemolytic anemia, eosinophilia, leukopenia, lymphocytosis, neutropenia, pancytopenia, thrombocytopenia

Nursing Considerations:

Assess I&O; notify MD for urine output < 30 cc/hr. Monitor lab studies for worsening renal or hepatic function or for blood dyscrasias. Monitor electrolytes if patient is on long-term therapy. Assess bowel status and notify MD for severe diarrhea. Assess IV site for infiltration and change as needed.

Precautions:

Use with caution in pregnancy (B), lactation, renal disease, or hypersensitivity to penicillin

Contraindications:

Hypersensitivity to cephalosporins, infants younger than 1 month

✤ ceftazidime

Trade: Ceptaz, Fortaz, Pentacef, Tazidime, Tazicef

Classification:

Antibiotic

Action:

- Inhibits cell wall synthesis of bacterial organism
- Changes cell wall osmolality and causes cell death

Clinical Application:

Used in the treatment of skin infections, upper and lower respiratory tract and urinary tract infections, septicemia, gonococcal and intra-abdominal infections and for meningitis. Used for gram positive bacteria (*S. pneumoniae, S. aureus, S. pyogenes*) and gram negative bacteria (*E. coli, P. mirabilis, Klebsiella, E. aerogenes, Citrobacter, Salmonella, Shigella, Acinetobacter, Neisseria, Serratia, and H. Influenzae*).

Dose:

Adult: 1g IV/IM q8-12h for 5-10 days; mix by diluting in 10 cc sterile H_2O for injection and give over 3-5 minutes; may be further diluted with 50-100 cc of NS or D_5W and run over 30 minutes

Child: 30-50 mg/kg/day IV; maximum of 6 g/day

Neonates: 30 mg/kg IV q12h

Side Effects:

CNS: Chills, dizziness, fever, headache, paresthesia, weakness

GI: Anorexia, increased AST, ALT, alkaline phosphatase, bilirubin, or LDH levels, bleeding, diarrhea, glossitis, nausea, pain, vomiting

GU: Increased BUN, candidiasis, nephrotoxicity, proteinuria, pruritus, renal failure, vaginitis

INTEG: Anaphylaxis, dermatitis, rash, urticaria

RESP: Dyspnea

HEMA: Agranulocytosis, anemia, hemolytic anemia, bleeding, eosinophilia, hypoprothrombinemia, leukopenia, lymphocytosis, pancytopenia, thrombocytopenia

Nursing Considerations:

Assess I&O; notify MD for urine output < 30 cc/hr. Monitor lab studies for worsening renal or hepatic function, or for blood dyscrasias. Assess bowel status and notify MD for severe diarrhea. Monitor IV site for infiltration and change as needed. Monitor for allergic reaction or bleeding.

Precautions:

Use with caution in patients with hypersensitivities to penicillin, pregnancy (B), lactation or in renal disease.

Contraindications:
Hypersensitivity to cephalosporins, infants younger than 1 month

---
✣ **ceftriaxone sodium**

Trade: Rocephin

Classification:
Antibiotic

Action:
- Changes osmotic pressure in cell wall causing bacterial cell death
- Inhibits cell wall synthesis of bacterial organism

Clinical Application:
Used in the treatment of infections involving the skin, bones, joints, lower respiratory tract, urinary tract, gonococcal infections, septicemia, meningitis, surgical prophylaxis, and for intra-abdominal infections. Used for gram positive organisms (*S. aureus, S. pyogenes, and S. pneumoniae*) and gram negative organisms (*E. coli, P. mirabilis, H. influenzae, Enterobacter, Salmonella, Shigella, Citrobacter, Neisseria, Serratia and Klebsiella*).

Dose:

Adult: 1-2 g IV/IM qd or in two divided doses for a total of 10-14 days; mix in 50-100 cc NSV, D_5W, or $D_{10}W$ and give over 30 min.

Child: 50-75 mg/kg/day IV/IM in divided doses q12h

Meningitis

Adult: 100 mg/kg/day IV/IM in divided doses q12h

Child: Same as adult

Side Effects:

CNS: Chills, dizziness, fever, headache, paresthesia, weakness

GI: Increased ALT, AST, alkaline phosphatase, bilirubin and LDH levels, abdominal pain, anorexia, bleeding, diarrhea, glossitis, nausea, pseudomembranous colitis, vomiting

GU: Increased BUN, candidiasis, proteinuria, pruritus, nephrotoxicity, renal failure, vaginitis

INTEG: Anaphylaxis, dermatitis, rash, urticaria

RESP: Dyspnea

HEMA: Agranulocytosis, anemia, hemolytic anemia, eosinophilia, lymphocytosis, leukopenia, neutropenia, pancytopenia, thrombocytopenia

Nursing Considerations:

Assess I&O; notify MD for urine output < 30 cc/hr. Monitor lab studies for renal or hepatic function decrease or blood dyscrasias. Monitor electrolytes for long-term therapy. Assess bowel status and notify MD for severe diarrhea. Monitor IV site for infiltration and change site as needed.

Precautions:

Use with caution in pregnancy (B), lactation, renal disease or hypersensitivity to penicillin

Contraindications:

Hypersensitivity to cephalosporins, infants younger than 1 month

✤ cefuroxime sodium

Trade: Kefurox, Zinacef

Classification:

Antibiotic

Action:

- Inhibits cell wall synthesis
- Changes osmotic pressure in bacterial cell causing organism death

Clinical Application:

Used for the treatment of infections involving the skin, lower respiratory tract, urinary tract, gonococcal infections, bacteremia, septicemia, and meningitis. Used for gram positive organisms (*S. aureus, S. Pyogenes, and S. pneumoniae*) and gram negative organisms (*E. coli, P. mirabilis, H. influenzae, Klebsiella, and Neisseria*).

Dose:

Adult: 750 mg-1.5 g IV/IM q8h for 5-10 days; mix with at least 10 cc of NS, sterile H_2O for injection, or D_5W and give over 3-5 min; may be further diluted in 50-100 cc of NS or D5W and given over 30 min; may also be added to 500-1000 cc of IV fluid and given over 6-24 hrs.

Severe infections

Adult: 1.5 g IV q6h; may give up to 3 g IV q8h for meningitis

Child > 3 mo: 50-100 mg/kg/day IV/IM; may give up to 200-240 mg/kg/day IV in divided doses for meningitis

Side Effects:

CNS: Chills, dizziness, fever, headache, paresthesia, weakness

GI: Increased ALT, AST, alkaline phosphatase, bilirubin and LDH levels, abdominal pain, anorexia, bleeding, diarrhea, glossitis, nausea, pseudomembranous colitis, vomiting

GU: Increased BUN, candidiasis, nephrotoxicity, proteinuria, pruritus, renal failure, vaginitis

INTEG: Anaphylaxis, dermatitis, inflammation to site, pain, rash, urticaria

RESP: Dyspnea

HEMA: Agranulocytosis, anemia, hemolytic anemia, eosinophilia, leukopenia, lymphocytosis, neutropenia, pancytopenia, thrombocytopenia

Nursing Considerations:

Assess I&O; notify MD for urine output < 30 cc/hr. Monitor lab studies for worsening renal or hepatic function or for blood dyscrasias. Monitor electrolytes if patient is on long-term therapy. Assess bowel status and notify MD for severe diarrhea. Assess IV site for infiltration and change site as needed.

Precautions:

Use with caution in pregnancy (B), lactation, renal disease, or hypersensitivity to penicillin.

Contraindications:

Hypersensitivity to cephalosporins, infants younger than 1 month.

✣ chloramphenicol

Trade: Chloramphenicol, Chloramphenicol Sodium Succinate, Chloromycetin Kapseals, Chloromycetin Sodium Succinate, Chloromycetin Palmitate,

Classification

Antibacterial, antirickettsial

Action:

- Binds to ribosomal subunit of organism
- Interferes with and inhibits protein synthesis

Clinical Application:

Used for the treatment of infections including mycoplasma, *H. Influenzae, S. typhi, Rickettsia,* and *Neisseria.*

Dose:

Adult: 50-100 mg/kg/day PO/IV in divided doses q6h for 10-14 days; maximum dose of 100 mg/kg/day; mix IV med with at least 10 cc sterile H_2O for injection of D_5W and give over at least 1 minute; may be further diluted in 50-100 cc of D_5W and given over 30 min.

Child: Same as adult

Neonates and premature infants: 25 mg/kg/day PO/IV in divided doses q6h.

Side Effects:

CNS: Confusion, depression, headache

CV: Cyanosis, vasomotor collapse, pallor

GI: Abdominal distention, abdominal pain, colitis, diarrhea, failure to feed, glossitis, nausea, pruritus to anal region, vomiting, xerostomia

RESP: Irregular respirations

INTEG: Dermatitis, itching, rash

EENT: Blindness, optic neuritis

HEMA: Anemia, aplastic anemia, bone marrow depression, granulocytopenia, leukopenia, thrombocytopenia

Nursing Considerations:

Assess VS; notify MD of abnormal respiratory status. Assess I&O; notify MD for urine output cc/hr. Monitor lab studies for renal function, liver function, and problems with blood studies. Drug levels should be done when used with liver or renal dysfunction patients.

Precautions:

Use with caution in pregnancy (C), infants, children, lactation, drug-induced bone marrow depression, hepatic or renal disease.

Contraindications:

Hypersensitivity, severe renal or hepatic disease, or with minor infections.

✤ clindamycin HCl

Trade: Cleocin HCl, Clindamycin HCl, Cleocin Phosphate, Clindamycin Phosphate

Classification:

Antibacterial macrolide

Action:

- Binds to subunit of ribosomes of bacterial organism
- Suppresses bacterial protein synthesis

Clinical Application:

Used in the treatment of infections caused by streptococci, staphylococci, *pneumonococci, Clostridium, Rickettsia, Actinomyces,* and *Peptococcus.*

Dose:

Adults: 300 mg IV/IM q6-12h for 10-14 days; mix with at least 50 cc of D_5W, or NS and give first dose over 30 min; should not exceed 1200 mg in 1 hr; maximum dose is 4800 mg/day

150-450 mg PO q6h

Child 1 mo: 15-40 mg/kg/day IV/IM in divided doses q6-8h;

8-25 mg/kg/day PO in divided doses q6-8h

PID

Adult: 600 mg IV qid with addition of gentamicin

Side Effects:

GI: Abdominal pain, anorexia, increased AST, ALT, alkaline phosphatase, and bilirubin levels, diarrhea, jaundice, nausea, pseudomembranous colitis, weight loss

GU: Urinary frequency, vaginitis

INTEG: Abscess at injection site, erythema, pain, pruritus, rash, urticaria

HEMA: Agranulocytosis, eosinophilia, leukopenia, thrombocytopenia

Nursing Considerations:

Assess VS and cardiopulmonary status; notify MD for wheezing, chest pain or tightness, or abnormal B/P or heart rates. Assess I&O; notify MD for urine output cc/hr. Assess bowel status and notify MD for severe diarrhea. Monitor lab studies for renal or hepatic dysfunction and for blood study abnormalities. Drug levels should be done on patients with renal or hepatic dysfunction. IM med should be given deeply with rotation of sites. PO med should be given with at least 8 ounces of water.

Precautions:

Use with caution in pregnancy (B), lactation, elderly, renal or hepatic disease, GI disease, or tartrazine sensitivity

Contraindications:

Hypersensitivity to this drug or lincomycin, infants younger than 1 month, or with ulcerative colitis

✤ chlorothiazide

Trade: Diuril, Diachlor, Diuril Sodium

Classification:

Diuretic

Action:

- Increases excretion of water, sodium, chloride, potassium, and magnesium by action on the distal tubule
- Diuretic and antihypertensive

Clinical Applications:

Used in the treatment of edema and for management of hypertension.

Dose:

Adult: 500 mg-2 g PO, IV qd in 2 divided doses; IV should be diluted with at least 10 cc of D_5W or 0.9% NS and given over at least 5 minutes.

Child < 6 mo: 10 mg/kg/day PO, IV, in 2 divided doses

Child > 6 mo: Up to 15 mg/kg/day PO, IV, in 2 divided doses

Side Effects:

CNS: Anxiety, confusion, depression, dizziness, drowsiness, fatigue, headache, paresthesias, restlessness, weakness

CV: Orthostatic hypotension, palpitations, irregular pulse, tachycardia, volume depletion

GI: Anorexia, constipation, cramps, diarrhea, GI irritation, hepatitis, nausea, pancreatitis, vomiting

GU: Glycosuria, frequency, impotence, polyuria, uremia

EENT: Blurred vision

INTEG: Fever, photosensitivity, purpura, rash, urticaria

MS: Leg cramps, weakness

META: Increased BUN and creatinine, hyperglycemia, hypomagnesemia, hyperuricemia, hypercalcemia, hypochloremia, hypokalemia, hypomagnesemia, hyponatremia, hypophosphatemia

HEMA: Aplastic anemia, hemolytic anemia, agranulocytosis, leukopenia, neutropenia, thrombocytopenia

RESP: Pulmonary edema, respiratory distress

Nursing Considerations:

Assess I&O; weigh daily. Observe for dependent edema to legs and sacrum. Maintain fluid balance. Monitor VS; orthostatic B/P readings, effect of exertion on respirations. Monitor electrolytes and renal lab studies for imbalances. Supplement potassium if level less than 3.0 mg/dl. PO drug should be given in the morning to prevent loss of sleep due to nocturia. Do not use sunscreen, especially those with PABA; instead use protective clothing against the sun.

Precautions:

Use with caution in COPD, diabetes, elderly, hypokalemia, hepatic or renal disease, gout, or lupus erythematosus

Contraindications:

Anuria, renal decompensation, pregnancy (D), lactation, or hypersensitivity to sulfonamide-derived drugs.

✤ chlorthalidone

Trade: Chlorthalidone, Hygroton, Hylidone, Thalitone

Classification:

Diuretic

Action:

- Increases excretion of sodium, water, chloride, potassium, magnesium, and bicarbonate in the cortical diluting segment of the ascending loop of Henle
- Antihypertensive and diuretic effects

Clinical Applications:

Used in the treatment of edema, hypertension, CHF, and nephrotic syndromes where diuresis is needed.

Dose:

Adult: 25-100 mg/day PO, or 100 mg PO every other day

Child: 2 mg/kg PO 3 times per week

Side Effects:

CNS: Anxiety, depression, dizziness, drowsiness, fatigue, headache, paresthesia, weakness

CV: Orthostatic hypotension, palpitations, irregular pulse, volume depletion

GI: Anorexia, constipation, cramps, diarrhea, GI irritation, hepatitis, nausea, pancreatitis, vomiting

GU: Frequency, glycosuria, polyuria, uremia

EENT: Blurred vision

INTEG: Fever, photosensitivity, purpura, rash, urticaria

HEMA: Aplastic anemia, hemolytic anemia, agranulocytosis, leukopenia, neutropenia, thrombocytopenia

META: Increased BUN and creatinine, hyperglycemia, hyperuremia, metabolic alkalosis, hypercalcemia, hypochloremia, hypokalemia, hypomagnesemia, hyponatremia

Nursing Considerations:

Assess I&O; weigh daily. Observe for edema changes. Maintain fluid balance. Monitor VS; orthostatic B/P readings, effect of exertion on respirations. Monitor lab studies for electrolyte imbalances, especially hypokalemia, renal studies, and for increased uric acid levels in patients with a history of gout. Supplement potassium if level 3.0 mg/dl. Assess for signs of digitalis toxicity if the patient is on digoxin. Administer drug in morning to avoid loss of sleep due to nocturia.

Precautions:
Use with caution hypokalemia, renal or hepatic disease, diabetes, gout, pregnancy (C), or elderly patients.

Contraindications:
Anuria, renal decompensation, lactation, or hypersensitivity to sulfonamide-derived drugs

---
✣ clonidine HCl

Trade: Catapres, Clonidine HCl

Classification:

Antihypertensive

Action:

- Decreases sympathetic cardioaccelerator and vasoconstrictor outflow from CNS
- Central-adrenergic stimulation
- Decreases B/P, pulse rate, peripheral vascular resistance and cardiac output
- Reduces plasma renin activity

Clinical Applications:

Used in the treatment of hypertension.

Dose:

Adult: 0.1 mg PO, transdermal patch qd; may increase by 0.1 mg/day or 0.2 mg/day until desired therapeutic response is achieved; usual range is 0.2-0.8 mg/day in divided doses. If patient is unable to swallow, pill may be given SL. Maximum 2.4 mg/day PO

Side Effects:

CNS: Anxiety, delirium, depression, drowsiness, fatigue, hallucinations, headache, insomnia, mental changes, nightmares, sedation, weakness

CV: AV block, bradycardia, CHF, EKG abnormalities, orthostatic hypotension, palpitations

GI: Constipation, dry mouth, malaise, nausea, vomiting

GU: Dysuria, gynecomastia, impotence, nocturia

EENT: Parotid pain, taste changes

INTEG: Alopecia, burning papules, edema, excoriation, hives, facial pallor, pruritus, rash

ENDO: Hyperglycemia, weight gain

MS: Leg cramps, muscular and joint pain

Nursing Considerations:

Assess VS: observe for postural hypotension. Assess I&O: observe for decrease in urinary output. Monitor lab studies for increasing BUN and creatinine, decreased platelets, and hypokalemia. Do not discontinue drug abruptly: taper over 2 weeks to prevent hypertension. Last dose should be taken before retiring each day. Avoid sunlight, or wear sunscreen as photosensitivity can occur. Do not use over-the-counter cough, cold or allergy medicines unless directed by MD.

Precautions:

Use cautiously with recent MI, severe coronary insufficiency, cerebral vascular disease, chronic renal failure, diabetes, thyroid disease, COPD, asthma, pregnancy (C), lactation, elderly, Raynaud's phenomenon, or with concurrent use of other antihypertensive drugs; may have increased bradycardia with concurrent use of β-blockers or cardiac glycosides.

Contraindications:

Hypersensitivity

✤ digoxin

Trade: Digoxin, Lanoxin

Classification:

Antidysrhythmic; cardiac glycoside

Action:

- Cardiac glycoside with positive inotropic and negative chronotropic effects
- Inhibits the sodium-potassium ATPase, making available more calcium for contractile proteins
- Increases cardiac contractility and cardiac output
- Decreases the speed of conduction through the AV node
- Decreases the heart rate

Clinical Applications:

Used for the treatment of heart failure, atrial fibrillation and flutter, or paroxysmal atrial tachycardia.

Dose:

Adult: 0.5 mg IV given over > 5 min, then 0.125-0.5 mg PO qd in divided doses q4-6h as needed; maintenance dose 0.125-0.625 mg PO qd

Elderly: 0.125 mg PO qd maintenance

Child > 2yr: 0.02-0.04 mg/kg PO divided q8h over 24 hr maintenance; 0.006-0.012 mg/kg PO qd in divided doses q12h; loading dose 0.015-0.035 mg/kg IV over 5 min; then convert to oral route.

Child 1 mo-2 yr: 0.03-0.05 mg/kg IV over 5 min in divided doses q4-8h; change to PO as soon as possible; 0.035-0.060 mg/kg PO divided in 3 doses over 24 hr; maintenance 0.01-0.02 mg/kg PO in divided doses q12h

Neonates: IV loading dose 0.02-0.03 mg/kg IV over > 5 min, in divided doses q4-8h; change to PO as soon as possible; loading dose 0.035 mg/kg PO in divided doses q8h over 24h; maintenance dose 0.01 mg/kg in divided doses q12h

Premature infants: 0.015-0.025 mg/kg IV divided in 3 doses over 24 hr, given over > 5 min; maintenance 0.003-0.009 mg/kg IV in divided doses q12h

Side Effects:

CNS: Apathy, confusion, disorientation, depression, hallucinations, headache, vertigo, weakness

CV: AV block, AV dissociation, bradycardia, dysrhythmias, hypotension, PR prolongation, PVCs, ST depression

GI: Abdominal pain, anorexia, diarrhea, nausea, vomiting

GU: Gynecomastia

EENT: Blurred vision, yellow vision, diplopia, photophobia

Nursing Considerations:

Continuous cardiac monitoring should be used during digitalization. Assess VS; assess apical pulse and notify MD if < 60 (or parameter set by MD) before giving med. Assess I&O; weigh daily. Replace potassium if level ≤ 3.0 mg/dl. Monitor lab studies for therapeutic drug levels (0.5-2 ng/ml), electrolyte imbalances or decreasing renal or liver function. Assume any dysrhythmia in children taking digoxin is a result of digoxin toxicity until proven otherwise.

Precautions:

Use with caution in renal disease, acute MI, AV block, severe respiratory disease, hypothyroidism, elderly, pregnancy (C), sinus nodal disease, lactation, or hypokalemia

Contraindications:

Ventricular fibrillation, advanced heart block

✤ disopyramide

Trade: Disopyramide, Norpace, Norpace CR

Classification:

Antidysrhythmic (Class IA)

Action:

- Decreases the rate of depolarization in phase 4
- Increases action potential duration and effective refractory period

- Reduces the disparity in refractory time between normal and infarcted myocardium

Clinical Applications:

Used for the treatment of atrial fibrillation or flutter and life-threatening ventricular dysrhythmias.

Dose:

Adult: 100-200 mg PO q6h; in renal dysfunction 100 mg PO q6h; Extended release 200 mg PO q12h; usual dosage 400-800 mg/day in divided doses

Child 12-18 yr: 6-15 mg/kg/day PO in divided doses q6h

Child 4-12 yr: 10-15 mg/kg/day PO in divided doses q6h

Child 1-4 yr: 10-12 mg/kg/day PO in divided doses q6h

Child <1 yr: 10-30 mg/kg/day PO in divided doses q6h

Side Effects:

CNS: Anxiety, depression, dizziness, fatigue, headache, insomnia, paresthesia, psychosis, syncope

CV: Angina, cardiac arrest, AV block, bradycardia, CHF, dysrhythmias, edema, hypotension, increased QRS, QT intervals, tachycardia

GI: Anorexia, constipation, diarrhea, dry mouth, flatulence, nausea, vomiting

GU: Hesitancy, impotence, urinary frequency, urinary retention, urinary urgency

EENT: Blurred vision, dry eyes, narrow-angle glaucoma, dry mouth, dry nose

INTEG: Pruritus, rash, urticaria

MS: Pain in extremities, weakness

RESP: Dyspnea

HEMA: Agranulocytosis, anemia, decreased hemoglobin and hematocrit, thrombocytopenia

META: Hypoglycemia, increased BUN and creatinine

Nursing Considerations:

Assess VS; notify MD for apical pulse rate < 60/min or hypotension. Assess I&O; weigh daily. Report weight gain; maintain fluid balance. Continuous cardiac monitoring/EKG for initiation of therapy. Notify MD for prolonged QT duration or widening QRS interval. Monitor lab studies for renal and liver function.

Precautions:

Use with caution in pregnancy (C), lactation, diabetes, renal or hepatic disease, myasthenia gravis, narrow-angle glaucoma, cardiomyopathy, conduction abnormalities, or children. Patients with atrial flutter/fibrillation should be digitalized prior to drug administration.

Contraindications:

Advanced heart block, uncompensated CHF, cardiogenic shock, sick sinus syndrome, or with prolonged QT intervals; do not administer within 48 hrs of verapamil

✣ dobutamine HCl

Trade: Dobutrex

Classification:

Adrenergic direct-acting β_1-agonist

Action:

- Direct-acting inotropic drug with mild chronotropic effects
- Stimulates β-1 and α-adrenergic receptors
- Mild vasodilation
- Increases myocardial contractility
- Increases B/P and stroke volume
- Increases cardiac output with less reflex increase in heart rate and B/P
- Increases oxygen requirements
- Increases renal and mesenteric blood flow
- Increases coronary blood flow by acting on β–1 receptors in the heart.
- Decreases pulmonary capillary wedge pressure and systemic vascular resistance
- Decreases peripheral vascular resistance slightly

Clinical Applications:

Used for short-term treatment of adults with cardiac decompensation, pulmonary congestion with low cardiac output, and in hypotensive patients for whom vasodilators cannot be utilized.

Dose:

Adult: Drip (500 mg/250 cc D5W or 0.9 % NS); start at 2.5 mcg/kg/min and titrate, trying to avoid increases in heart rate of more than 10% from original value; maximum dose is 40 µg/kg/min; usual dose range is 2.5-10 µg/kg/min.

Side Effects:

CNS: Anxiety, dizziness, fatigue, headache, paresthesias

CV: Chest pain, dysrhythmias, hypertension, palpitations, shortness of breath, tachycardia.

GI: Nausea, vomiting

MS: Leg cramps

INTEG: Inflammation of site, phlebitis

Nursing Considerations:

Patient's heart rhythm should be continuously monitored during administration. Hemodynamic monitoring, when possible, should be done with titration of drug based on parameters set by physician. B/P and pulse should be monitored q5-15 min during active titration. I&O q1-2 hrs. Solution should be changed at least q24 hrs. Aim is for maximum physiological response with minimal amount of medicine.

Precautions:

Use with caution in pre-existing hypertension or acute MI. Do not give with bicarbonate solutions, or with any other drug or solution.

Contraindications:

Ventricular tachycardia or IHSS

✣   dopamine HCl

Trade: Dopamine HCl, Intropin

Classification:

Agonist

Action:

- Positive inotropic and chronotropic effects
- Causes a release of norepinephrine from storage sites
- Increases cardiac output
- Improves renal blood flow and causes vasodilation of renal, mesenteric and cerebral arteries at low doses (< 2 µg/kg/min)
- Stimulates β-1 and α-adrenergic receptors depending on dose range
- Increases myocardial contractility and heart rate at intermediate doses (2-10 µg/kg/min) (predominately β-1 stimulation)
- Vasoconstriction occurs with rates > 20 µg/kg/min (predominately α-stimulation)
- Modestly increases systemic vascular resistance
- Increases myocardial contractility and heart rate at intermediate doses (2-10 µg/kg/min)
- Increases pulmonary capillary wedge pressure and preload
- May induce or worsen pulmonary congestion

Clinical Applications:

Used for the treatment of all forms of shock (except hypovolemic), to improve renal perfusion and for correction of hypotension.

Dose:

Adult: Drip (400 mg/250 cc D5W, 0.9% NS, D5W 0.9% NS, D5W. 45% NaCl, D5 0.9% NS, D5 RL or RL) Start at 2-5 µg/kg/min and titrate to obtain the desired hemodynamic benefit with the lowest amount of medicine; maximum dose 20 µg/kg/min.

Side Effects:

CNS: Headache

CV: Chest pain, ectopy, hypertension, palpitations, tachycardia, shortness of breath, peripheral perfusion decrease

GI: Nausea, vomiting, diarrhea

GU: Azotemia

INTEG: Gangrene, tissue necrosis and sloughing with infiltration

Nursing Considerations:

Continuous cardiac monitoring should be used during administration. Hemodynamic monitoring, when possible, should be done with titration of drug based on parameters set by physician. Aim is for maximum effect with minimum amount of medicine necessary. B/P and pulse should be monitored q5-15 min during active titration. I&O q1-2 hrs. Avoid hypovolemia. If extravasation occurs, infiltrate area with 5-10 mg phentolamine and 10-15 cc NS to decrease tissue necrosis and sloughing. Observe for vasoconstrictor activity if disproportionate rise in diastolic B/P seen.

Precautions:

Occlusive vascular disease, pregnancy (C), lactation, or children; effects potentiated with MAO inhibitors, bretylium, phenytoin sodium, or barbiturates; drug is incompatible with alkaline solutions

Contraindications:

Use with caution in patients with pheochromocytoma, hypersensitivity to metabisulfites, or ventricular dysrhythmias

---

✤ epinephrine

Trade: Adrenalin Chloride, Adrenalin Chloride Solution, Epinephrine Pediatric

Classification:

Sympathomimetic amine

Action:

- Naturally occurring catecholamine with α and β-adrenergic activity
- Increases systemic vascular resistance, B/P, and heart rate
- Large doses cause vasoconstriction; small doses cause vasodilation by β-2 receptor activity
- Increases cerebral and coronary blood flow
- Increases myocardial contraction

- Increases automaticity
- Reduces congestion and edema in lungs
- Makes ventricular fibrillation more susceptible to DC countershock

Clinical Applications:

Used in ventricular fibrillation, pulseless ventricular tachycardia, asystole, electromechanical dissociation, PEA, syncope due to heart block, anaphylaxis, bronchospasm, allergic reactions and acute asthmatic episodes.

Dose:

Adult: 0.5 to 1.0 mg of 1:10,000 solution IV, ETT every 5 min as needed

Child: 5-10 µg, IV, ETT q5 min prn, may use drip of 0.1 mg/kg/min after initial dose; ETT dose must be diluted with 10 cc NS.

Allergic Reaction:

Adult: 0.1-0.5 ml of 1:1000 solution IM, SQ q10-15 min as needed; 0.1-0.25 ml of 1:1000 solution IV

Child: 0.01 ml of 1:1000 solution/kg SQ q20 min to 4 hrs as needed

Side Effects:

CNS: Anxiety, confusion, cerebral hemorrhage, dizziness, hallucinations, headache, insomnia, tremors

CV: Dysrhythmias, hypertension, palpitations, tachycardia, shortness of breath

GI: Anorexia, nausea, vomiting

Nursing Considerations:

Continuous cardiac monitoring should be used during administration. B/P and pulse q5 min after IV, ET routes. IM injections should not be given in the buttocks. Medications given ETT *must* be diluted in 10 cc NS.

Precautions:

Use with caution in pregnancy (C). Do not give in conjunction with alkaline solutions or MAO inhibitors.

Contraindications:

Narrow angle glaucoma, hypertension, concurrent use of isoproterenol

---

✣ erythromycin

Trade: E-Base, E-Mycin, Eryc, Ery-Tab, Erythromycin, Erythromycin Base, Erythromycin Filmtabs, PCE Dispertab, Erythromycin Estolate, Ilosone, E.E.S. 400, Eryped, Erythromycin Ethylsuccinate, Erythromycin Lactobionate, Ilotycin Gluceptate

Classification:

Antibacterial

Action:

- Binds to subunits of ribosome of bacterial organism;
- Suppresses protein synthesis of organism

Clinical Application:

Used in the treatment of infections involving the skin, soft tissue, respiratory tract, and those infections caused by *D. pneumoniae, M. pneumoniae, B. pertussis, B. burgdorferi, N. gonorrhoeae, C. diphtheriae, L. monocytogenes,* Legionnaire's disease, *H. influenzae,* and syphilis.

Dose

Soft Tissue Infections

Adult: 15-20 mg/kg/day IV; mix with at least 10 cc sterile H2O for injection and dilute in 80-250 cc NS or RL and give over 30 min. to 1 hour; may be mixed as a continuous infusion over 6 hours.

250-500 mg PO q6h; or 400-800 mg PO q6h

Child: 15-20 mg/kg/day IV in divided doses q4-6h

30-50 mg/kg/day PO in divided doses q6h

Gonorrhea/PID

Adult: 500 mg IV q6h for 3 days, then change to 250-400 mg PO q6h for 1 week

Syphilis

Adult: 20 g PO in divided doses over 15 days

Chlamydia

Adult: 500 mg PO q6h for 1 week or 250 mg PO qid for 2 weeks

Infant: 50 mg/kg/day in 4 divided doses for 3 weeks or more

Newborn: 50 mg/kg/day in 4 divided doses for 2 weeks or more

Intestinal Amebiasis

Adult: 250 mg PO q6h for 10-14 days

Child: 30-50 mg/kg/day PO in divided doses q6h for 10-14 days

Side Effects:

GI: Abdominal pain, anorexia, diarrhea, heartburn, hepatotoxicity, nausea, pruritus in anal region, vomiting

GU: Moniliasis, vaginitis

INTEG: Pruritus, rash, thrombophlebitis with IV use

EENT: Hearing loss, tinnitus

Nursing considerations:

Assess VS; notify MD for wheezing or respiratory difficulty. Assess I&O; notify MD for urine output < 30 cc/hr or hematuria. Monitor lab studies for renal and hepatic dysfunction. PO med should not be taken with fruit juice.

Precautions:

Use with caution in pregnancy (C), lactation, or hepatic disease

Contraindications:

Hypersensitivity

✣ esmolol HCl

Trade: Brevibloc

Classification:

β–Adrenergic blocker

Action:

- Competitively blocks stimulation of β1-adrenergic receptors in the myocardium
- Produces negative chronotropic and inotropic activity
- Decreases rate of SA node discharge and increases recovery time
- Slows conduction of AV node
- Decreases heart rate and myocardial oxygen consumption
- Decrease renin-aldosterone-angiotensin system at high doses.
- Slightly inhibits β-2 receptors in bronchial system

Dose:

Adult: Drip of 2.5 g/250 cc D5W, D5RL, D5NS, RL or NS) IV with 500 µg/kg/min loading dose given over 1 min; maintenance dose of 50 µg/kg/min, for 4 min (maximum dose 300 µg/kg/min), titrate for desired therapeutic effect. If necessary, the loading dose may be repeated, with the maintenance dose increased to 100 µg/kg/min

Side Effects:

CNS: Agitation, anxiety, asthenia, confusion, dizziness, fatigue, fever, headache, paresthesias, seizures, syncope

CV: AV block, bradycardia, chest pain, CHF, conduction disturbances, hypotension, peripheral ischemia

GI: Abdominal discomfort, anorexia, bloating, constipation, flatulence, gastric pain, heartburn, nausea, vomiting

GU: Dysuria, impotence, urinary retention

INTEG: Alopecia, burning, discoloration, dry skin, edema, erythema, fever, flushing, induration or inflammation at site, local skin necrosis, pallor, pruritus, rash

RESP: Bronchospasm, nasal congestion, dyspnea, rales, wheezing

Nursing Considerations:

Continuous cardiac monitoring must be used. Notify MD of AV block or rhythm disturbances. Assess VS: B/P q1-5 min during initial titration, then q15 min until stable, then q4h. Notify MD for systolic B/P <100 or diastolic <60 or pulse <60/min. Assess I&O: weigh daily; maintain fluid balance. Notify MD for urine output 30 cc/hr. Observe skin turgor and mucous membranes for hydration status. Assess for edema to lower extremities. No over-the-counter cough, cold or allergy medications without MD approval. Monitor lab studies for renal and liver function.

Precautions:

Use with caution in hypotension, pregnancy (C), lactation, peripheral vascular disease, diabetes, hypoglycemia, thyrotoxicosis, or impaired renal function. Incompatible with alkaline solutions or any other drug before dilution.

Contraindications:

Advanced heart block, cardiac failure, CHF, cardiogenic shock, or children.

✣ ethacrynic acid

Trade: Edecrin, Edecrin Sodium

Classification:

Loop diuretic

Action:

- Inhibits reabsorption of sodium, chloride, and water in the ascending loop of Henle with a weak diuretic effect in the proximal and distal tubules
- Potent diuretic

Clinical Applications:

Used in the treatment of pulmonary edema as well as the edema in CHF, liver disease, and nephrotic syndrome.

Dose:

Adult: 0.5-1.0 mg/kg IV (Usual dose 50 mg) after diluting with 50 cc of NaCl given at rate no faster than 10 mg/min. May be infused as an intermittent infusion to the lowest port on the IV tubing over 30 min; 50-200 mg PO qd; occasional cases may need 200 mg PO bid

Child: 25 mg PO qd; increase by 25 mg/day until therapeutic effect achieved

Side Effects:

CNS: Apprehension, confusion, fatigue, headache, vertigo, weakness

CV: Chest pain, circulatory collapse, EKG changes, hypotension

GI: Abdominal pain, anorexia, cramps, severe diarrhea, dry mouth, GI bleeding, jaundice, nausea, acute pancreatitis, upset stomach, vomiting

GU: Glycosuria, polyuria, renal failure

EENT: Blurred vision, ear pain, loss of hearing, tinnitus

INTEG: Photosensitivity, pruritus, purpura, rash, Stevens-Johnson syndrome, sweating

MS: Arthritis, cramps

HEMA: Agranulocytosis, leukopenia, neutropenia, thrombocytopenia

ENDO: Decreased glucose tolerance, hyperglycemia, hyperuricemia, hypochloremic alkalosis, hypocalcemia, hypokalemia, hypomagnesemia, hyponatremia

Nursing Considerations:

Assess I&O; weigh daily. Observe for improvement in edema. Maintain fluid balance. If warranted, increase fluid intake to 2-3 L/day. Potassium replacement should occur with levels < 3.0 mg/dl. If azotemia or oliguria occurs, drug may need to be discontinued. Assess VS; observe for postural hypotension and dyspnea with exertion. Monitor lab studies for electrolyte imbalances, increased levels of uric acid, or change in ABGs. Administer med in the morning to prevent nocturia. IV injection may be very painful and can cause thrombophlebitis.

Precautions:

Use with caution in ascites, severe renal disease, pregnancy (D), dehydration and hypoproteinemia. Drug may potentiate effects of anticoagulant, warfarin. May cause transient deafness with too rapid IV injection.

Contraindications:

Hypersensitivity to sulfonamides, anuria, hypovolemia, lactation, infants, and in electrolyte depletion.

✤ flecainide acetate

Trade: Tambocor

Classification:

Antidysrhythmic (Class IC)

Action:

- Decreases conduction in all parts of the heart, with greatest effect on His-Purkinje system, which stabilizes the cardiac membrane
- Decreases ejection fraction
- Increases endocardial pacing thresholds
- Increases sinus node recovery time

Clinical Applications:

Used for treatment of severe or sustained ventricular dysrhythmias, and for the prevention of paroxysmal supraventricular tachydysrhythmias in patients without structural heart disease.

Dose:

Adult: 50-100 mg PO q12h, may increase by 50 mg q12h every 4 days until desired response achieved (maximum dose is 300-400 mg/day)

Side Effects:

CNS: Anxiety, asthenia, ataxia, confusion, depression, dizziness, fatigue, flushing, headache, irritability, malaise, paresthesias, restlessness, somnolence, tremors

CV: Angina, AV block, arrest, bradycardia, cardiovascular collapse, CHF, dysrhythmias, hypertension, hypotension, ventricular ectopy, fatal ventricular tachycardia

GI: Abdominal pain, anorexia, constipation, flatulence, jaundice, nausea, taste changes, vomiting

GU: Impotence, decreased libido, polyuria, urinary retention

EENT: Dry mouth, eye pain, hearing loss, photophobia, tinnitus, visual disturbances

INTEG: Edema, rash, swelling, urticaria

RESP: Bronchospasm, dyspnea, respiratory depression

HEMA: Blood dyscrasias, leukopenia, thrombocytopenia

Nursing Considerations:

Assess VS: notify MD of changes in B/P, tachypnea, elevated temperature, or increased pulse. Assess for rales or respiratory depression. Cardiac monitoring recommended for initiation of therapy. Monitor lab studies for electrolyte imbalances.

Precautions:

Use with caution in pregnancy (C), lactation, children, renal or liver disease, CHF, respiratory depression, myasthenia gravis, sick sinus syndrome or myocardial dysfunction.

Contraindications:

Recent MI, chronic atrial fibrillation, advanced heart block, cardiogenic shock and non-life-threatening dysrhythmias

---

✣ fluconazole

Trade: Diflucan

Classification:

Antifungal

Action:

- Damages phospholipids in fungal membrane
- Inhibits biosynthesis of ergosterol

Clinical Application:

Used for the treatment of chronic mucocutaneous candidiasis, oropharyngeal candidiasis with HIV patients, urinary candidiasis and cryptococcal meningitis.

Dose:

Serious Fungal Infections

Adult: 50-400 mg IV initially, then 200 mg IV qd for 4 weeks; mix according to package insert directions and give at rate no faster than 200 mg/hr

PO 50-400 mg initially, then 200 mg PO qd for 4 weeks

Oropharyngeal Candidiasis

Adult: 200 mg initially, then 100 mg PO qd for 2 weeks

Vaginal Candidiasis

Adult: 150 mg PO as a single dose

Side Effects:

CNS: Seizures

GI: Increased ALT and AST levels, cramping, diarrhea, flatus, nausea, vomiting

INTEG: Stevens-Johnson syndrome

Nursing Considerations:

Assess VS q15-30 minutes during initial infusion; note changes in heart rate and blood pressure. Assess I&O; notify MD for urine output 30cc/hr; weigh daily and notify MD for weight gain of 2 5 pounds/week or edema. Do not use plastic containers in connections with IV administration; use an in-line filter. Observe site for extravasation and necrosis at least q2h. Monitor lab studies for worsening renal or hepatic dysfunction. Incompatible with other drugs in solution or syringe.

Precautions:

Use with caution in pregnancy (B) or renal disease. Concurrent use with phenytoin may increase concentrations of phenytoin.

Contraindications:

Hypersensitivity

✣ furosemide

Trade: Fumide, Furomide M.D., Furosemide, Lasix, Luramide

Classification:

Loop diuretic

Action:

- Inhibits reabsorption of sodium and chloride at the proximal and distal tubules, and at the proximal end of the ascending loop of Henle
- Potent diuretic

Clinical Applications:

Used in the treatment of pulmonary edema and the edema of CHF, liver disease, nephrotic syndrome, ascites, and hypertension.

Dose:

Pulmonary Edema

Adult: 40 mg IV over 2 min, followed by 40-80 mg IV after 1 hr if needed, may be given as IV infusion in D_5W or 0.9% NS at a rate no faster than 4 mg/min.

Edema

Adult: 20-40 mg IM/IV given over 1-2 min, increase by 20 mg/2 hrs until desired response achieved; 20-80 mg/day PO in the morning; may give another dose in 6 hours, maximum dose of 600 mg/day PO

Child: 2 mg/kg PO/IM/IV; may increase by 1-2 mg/kg per 6-8 hrs up to a maximum of 6 mg/kg/day.

Side Effects:

CNS: Fatigue, headache, paresthesias, vertigo, weakness

CV: Chest pain, circulatory collapse, EKG changes, orthostatic hypotension

GI: Anorexia, cramps, diarrhea, dry mouth, oral and gastric irritations, nausea, pancreatitis, vomiting

GU: Glycosuria, polyuria, renal failure, urinary bladder spasms

EENT: Blurred vision, ear pain, loss of hearing, tinnitus

INTEG: Photosensitivity, pruritus, purpura, rash, Stevens-Johnson syndrome, sweating

MS: Muscular cramps

HEMA: Anemia, agranulocytosis, leukopenia, neutropenia, thrombocytopenia

ENDO: Hyperglycemia, hyperuricemia, hypocalcemia, hypochloremic alkalosis, hypokalemia, hypomagnesemia, hyponatremia, metabolic alkalosis

Nursing Considerations:

Assess I&O; weigh daily. Monitor hydration with skin turgor and mucous membranes. Observe for decreased edema. Maintain fluid balance. Assess VS: observe for dyspnea on exertion or postural hypotension. Potassium replacement should occur for < 3.0 mg/dl level. Monitor lab studies for electrolyte imbalances, worsening renal function studies, ABG changes or uric acid level changes. Administer PO med in the morning to avoid nocturia.

Precautions:

Use with caution in dehydration, severe renal disease, pregnancy (C), or diabetes. Hearing may be affected with high doses or rapid IV administration.

Contraindications:

Hypersensitivity to sulfonamides, anuria, hypovolemia, lactation, electrolyte depletion and infants

✣ gentamicin sulfate

Trade: Apogen, Garamycin, Gentamicin Sulfate, Jenamicin

Classification:

Antibiotic

Action:

- Binds to ribosome and changes genetic coding causing bacterial death

Clinical Application:

Used for the treatment of severe systemic infections involving the central nervous system, skin, soft tissues, bones, urinary tract, respiratory and GI tracts. Useful for *P. aeruginosa, Klebsiella, Proteus, E. coli, Enterobacter, Proteus, Citrobacter, Salmonella, Shigella,* and *Staphylococcus.*

Dose:

Adult: 3-5 mg/kg/day in 3 divided doses q8h; mixed in 50-200 cc D_5W or NS and given over 30 min-2 hours

3 mg/kg/day IM in divided doses q8h

Intrathecal: 4-8 mgqd

Child: 2-2.5 mg/kg IV/IM q8h

Neonates and infants: 2.5 mg/kg IV/IM q8h

Neonates < 1 wk: 2.5 mg IV/IM q12h

Infants and children >3 months: intrathecal 1-2 mg qd

CNS: Confusion, convulsions, dizziness, depression, neurotoxicity, numbness, tremors, muscle twitching, vertigo

CV: Hypertension, hypotension, palpitations

GI: Increased ALT, AST, or bilirubin levels, anorexia, hepatomegaly, hepatic necrosis, nausea, splenomegaly, vomiting

GU: Azotemia, hematuria, nephrotoxicity, renal damage and failure

EENT: Deafness, ototoxicity, tinnitus, visual disturbances

INTEG: Alopecia, burning, dermatitis, rash, urticaria

HEMA: Agranulocytosis, anemia, eosinophilia, leukopenia, thrombocytopenia

Nursing Considerations:

Assess VS; observe for hypotensive changes or heart rate changes. Assess I&O; weigh daily. Maintain fluid balance. Encourage fluids up to 3 L/day if warranted. Assess hydration status with skin turgor and mucous membranes. Notify MD for urine output < 30 cc/hr. Monitor lab studies for therapeutic levels [peak 4-10 µg/ml, trough 1-2 µg/ml] and for deterioration of renal status. Monitor IV site for infiltration and change site as needed. Assess for hearing deficit.

Precautions:

Use with caution in pregnancy (C), neonates, myasthenia gravis, Parkinson's disease, mild renal disease, lactation and the elderly.

Contraindications:

Hypersensitivity, severe renal disease

✤ hydralazine HCl

Trade: Alazine, Apresoline, Hydralazine HCl

Classification:

Antihypertensive, direct-acting peripheral vasodilator

Action:

- Relaxes vascular smooth muscle

- Reduces B/P with reflex increases in heart rate, stroke volume, and cardiac output
- Decreases peripheral vascular resistance
- Increases plasma renin activity

Clinical Applications:

Used in essential hypertension.

Dose:

Adult: 20-40 mg bolus given IV at the rate of 10 mg/min q4-6h prn: begin PO form as soon as feasible.

20-40 mg IM q4-6h prn: begin PO form as soon as feasible.

10 mg PO qid for 2-4 days, then 25 mg for the rest of the first week, then 50 mg qid or as needed to achieve desired response; maximum dose is 300 mg/day

Child: 0.1-0.2 mg/kg IV bolus q4-6h prn

0.1-0.2 mg/kg IM q4-6h prn

0.75 mg/kg qd PO; 0.75-3 mg/kg/day in 4 divided doses, with a maximum of 7.5 mg/kg/day

Side Effects:

CNS: Anxiety, depression, dizziness, headache, peripheral neuritis, tremors

CV: Angina, edema, dysrhythmias, rebound hypertension, palpitations, shock, reflex tachycardia

GI: Anorexia, constipation, diarrhea, nausea, vomiting

GU: Impotence, sodium and water retention, urinary retention

EENT: Nasal congestion, conjunctivitis

INTEG: Pruritus, rash

MS: Arthralgia, muscular cramps

HEMA: Agranulocytosis, anemia, leukopenia, splenomegaly

OTHER: Lupus-like symptoms, weight gain

Nursing Considerations:

Assess VS: B/P q5-10 minutes for 2 hrs, q1h for 4 hours, then q4h. Assess heart rate and jugular vein distention q4h. Observe for postural hypotension or dyspnea. After IV administration, patient should be kept in supine position for at least 1 hr. Assess I&O; weigh daily. Maintain fluid balance. Observe skin turgor and mucous membranes for hydration. LE prep and ANA titer should be done prior to administration and periodically during course of treatment. Monitor lab studies for electrolyte imbalances, changes in renal function studies, or CBC, ABG changes, or uric acid level changes. Administer PO med in the morning to avoid nocturia.

Precautions:

Use with caution in pregnancy (C), CVA, or advanced renal disease

Contraindications:

Coronary artery disease, mitral valvular rheumatic heart disease, or rheumatic heart disease

✥ imipenem/cilastatin

Trade: Primaxin IV

Classification:

Anti-infective

Action:

- Interferes with replication of cells walls of organism
- Causes changes in osmotic pressure in the cell leading to cell explosion and death for organism

Clinical Application:

Used in the treatment of severe infections caused by gram negative organisms (*Acinetobacter, Campylobacter, E. coli, P. aeruginosa, Proteus, Salmonella, Serratia, shigella*) and gram positive organisms (*enterococcus, betahemolytic streptococcus, S. aureus, S. pneumoniae*), anaerobes (*bacteroides, clostridium, actinomyces*), bacterial septicemia, bone and joint infections, skin infections, respiratory tract infections, urinary tract infections, intra-abdominal or gynecological infections, and endocarditis.

Dosage:

Adult: 250-500 mg in 100 cc D_5W or NS IV over 30 minutes 16 hrs; may require 1 g over 40-60 minutes q6h; maximum 50 mg/kg/day or 4 g/day [whichever is lowest]

500-750 mg IM q12h; should be prepared with lidocaine 1%

Side Effects:

CNS: Confusion, dizziness, fever, headache, paresthesia, seizures, somnolence, weakness

CV: Hypotension, palpitations, tachycardia

GI: Anuria, oliguria, polyuria, increased BUN and creatinine

EENT: Glossitis

INTEG: Edema, erythematous site, flushing, pain at site, phlebitis, pruritus, rash

RESP: Dyspnea, hyperventilation

Nursing Considerations:

Assess VS. Monitor for allergic reactions. Assess bowel status and notify MD for severe diarrhea. Do not administer by IV bolus.

Precautions

Use with caution in pregnancy (C), lactation, elderly, hypersensitivity to penicillin, seizures, children and with renal disease.

Contraindications:

Hypersensitivity, hypersensitivity to local anesthetics of the amide type with IM administration

✢ isoproterenol HCl

Trade: Dispos-a-Med Isoproterenol HCl, Isuprel, Isoproterenol HCl, Isuprel Glossets, Isuprel Mistometer, Medihaler-Iso, Norisoprine Aerotrol

Classification:
Adrenergic

Action:
- Relaxes bronchial smooth muscles and dilates bronchi by increasing levels of cAMP
- Synthetic sympathomimetic amine with β-adrenergic receptor activity which causes increased contractility
- Increases cardiac output, heart rate, and systolic blood pressure
- Increases myocardial oxygen requirement
- May induce or exacerbate myocardial ischemia
- Decreases systemic vascular resistance, peripheral vascular resistance, and diastolic blood pressure

Clinical Applications:

Used for the temporary control of hemodynamically compromised and atropine-refractory bradyarrhythmias in a patient who has a pulse, for refractory torsades de pointes, bronchospasm, and as an adjunct with hypovolemia and septic shock.

Dose:

Shock

Adult: Drip (2 mg of 1:5000 solution/500 cc D_5W), start at 0.5-5 μg/min and titrate until heart rate is 60/min, B/P stable, and urine output adequate

Child: 0.1 μg/kg/min; usual range 0.1 to 1.0 μg/kg/min

Dysrhythmias

Adult: 0.02-0.06 mg of 1:5000 solution in 10 cc NS IV over 1 min then 0.01-0.2 mg or 5 μg/min

Adult: 0.2 mg IM, then 0.02-1 mg IM prn

Child: 0.01-0.03 mg IV, 0.1 mg IM prn

Asthma/bronchospasm

Adult: 10-20 mg SL q6-8h

Inhaler: 1 puff, may repeat after 2-5 min, with maintenance of 1-2 puffs 4-6 times per day prn

Child: 5-10 mg SL q6-8h

Inhaler: 1 puff, may repeat after 2-5 min, with maintenance of 1-2 puffs 4-6 times per day prn

Side Effects:

CNS: Anxiety, dizziness, headache, insomnia, tremors

CV: Angina, hypotension, hypertension, palpitations, tachycardia, ventricular tachycardia, ventricular fibrillation

GI: Nausea, vomiting

RESP: Bronchospasm, bronchial irritation, edema

INTEG: Flushing, sweating

OTHER: Hyperglycemia

Nursing Considerations:

Continuous cardiac monitoring must be used with IV administration. Infusion rate should be titrated to keep heart rate < 110-130/min. Assess VS and lung sounds. Assess I&O; weigh daily. Monitor lab studies, especially ABGs, for acid base problems. Isuprel should not be administered *simultaneously* with epinephrine, which could possibly cause dysrhythmias.

Precautions:

Use with caution in pregnancy (C) or potent inhalation anesthetics. Do not give in conjunction with alkaline solutions. Avoid use in patients with ischemic heart disease, diabetes or hyperthyroidism.

Contraindications:

Tachydysrhythmias, digitalis-toxicity-induced heart block or tachycardia, and angina

❖ kanamycin sulfate

Trade: Kanamycin Sulfate, Kantrex

Classification

Antibiotic

Action:

- Binds to ribosomal subunit
- Interferes with protein synthesis in bacterial organism
- Alters peptide sequencing in protein chain causing organism death

Clinical Application:

Used in the treatment for severe infections involving the skin, bones, respiratory tract, GI tract, urinary tract, CNS, and soft tissues. Used for infections caused by *Shigella, H. influenzae, E. coli, Enterobacter, Acinetobacter, Proteus, N. gonorrhoeae, S. marcescens, Staphylococcus* and *K. pneumoniae*. Used as an adjunct with hepatic coma, peritonitis and pre- and intra-operatively with contamination of bowel.

Dosage:

Severe Infections

Adult: 15 mg/kg/day IV in divided doses q8-12h; mix with 100 cc D_5W, D_5NS, or NS per 500 mg of medication and give over at least 30 minutes; maximum dose is 1.5 g/day

15 mg/kg/day IM in divided doses q8-12h; maximum dose is 1.5 g/day

Irrigation solution not to exceed 1.5 g/day

Child: same as adult

Hepatic Coma

Adult: 8-12 g/day individed doses

Preoperative Bowel Prep

Adult: 1 g PO qh for 4 doses, then q6h for 36-72 hrs prior to surgery

Side Effects:

CNS: Confusion, convulsions, depression, neurotoxicity, numbness, tremors, muscle twitching

CV: Hypotension

GI: Increased AST, ALT, and bilirubin levels, anorexia, hepatic necrosis, nausea, splenomegaly, vomiting

GU: Azotemia, hematuria, nephrotoxicity, oliguria, renal failure or damage

RESP: Respiratory depression

INTEG: Alopecia, burning, dermatitis, rash, urticaria

EENT: Deafness, dizziness, ototoxicity, tinnitus, vertigo, visual disturbances

HEMA: Agranulocytosis, anemia, eosinophilia, leukopenia, thrombocytopenia

Nursing Considerations:

Assess VS; observe for hypotension or changes in heart rate. Assess I&O; notify MD for urine output < 30 cc/hr; weigh daily. Maintain fluid hydration; encourage fluid intake of 2-3 L/day if warranted. Monitor IV site for infiltration and change site as needed. Drug levels should be drawn periodically; peak levels should be drawn 60 minutes after IV infusion [< 30 mEq/ml] and trough level just prior to dose [5-10 mEq/ml]. Give IM medication in large muscle and rotate sites. Concurrent use of penicillin should be alternated whereby the penicillin is given at least 1 hour prior to or after kanamycin.

Precautions:

Use with caution in pregnancy (D), lactation, neonates, hearing dysfunction, myasthenia gravis, mild renal disease, or Parkinson's disease.

Contraindications:

Hypersensitivity, severe renal disease or bowel obstruction

✣ labetalol

Trade: Normodyne, Trandate

Classification:

Antihypertensive

Action:

- Non-selective β-blocker
- Selective α-1 blocker
- Depresses plasma renin secretion
- Produces falls in blood pressure without reflex tachycardia or significant reduction in heart rate

Clinical Applications:

Used in the treatment of severe hypertension.

Dose:

Adult: 20 mg IV bolus given over 2 min; may repeat 40-80 mg IV q10 min with a maximum of 300 mg/day.

Drip (200 mg/160 cc D$_5$W, NS, RL, D$_5$RL, D$_5$ ½ NS, D$_5$NS) to run at 2 ml/min (2 mg/min); infusion should be stopped after the desired therapeutic response is achieved; may be repeated q6-8 hrs prn.

100 mg PO bid; may increase up to 200 mg PO bid after 2 days, and may increase q1-3d: maximum dose of 1200-2400 mg/day

Side Effects:

CNS: Anxiety, catatonia, depression, dizziness, drowsiness, fatigue, headache, lethargy, mental changes, nightmares, paresthesia

CV: AV block, bradycardia, chest pain, CHF, orthostatic hypotension, ventricular dysrhythmias

GI: Diarrhea, nausea, vomiting

GU: Dysuria, impotence

RESP: Bronchospasm, dyspnea, wheezing

EENT: Dry, burning eyes, sore throat, tinnitus, visual changes, taste distortion

INTEG: Alopecia, fever, pruritus, rash, urticaria

HEMA: Agranulocytosis, purpura, thrombocytopenia

Nursing Considerations:

Cardiac monitoring should be used during IV administration. Assess I&O; weigh daily. Observe for edema. Maintain fluid balance and assess mucous membranes and skin turgor for hydration. Assess VS; B/P q5-10 minutes during active titration of drug. Observe for hypotension. After IV medication administration, keep patient supine for 3 hours. Obtain baseline renal and liver function studies prior to administration. Do not use over-the-counter cold, cough, allergy, nasal decongestants without MD approval. Do not discontinue PO medications abruptly—taper over 2 weeks.

Precautions:

Use with caution in major surgery, pregnancy (C), lactation, diabetes, renal or thyroid disease, COPD, coronary artery disease, or nonallergic bronchospasm. Incompatible with alkaline solutions or other drugs in syringe.

Contraindications:

Hypersensitivity to ß-blockers, cardiogenic shock, advanced heart block, sinus bradycardia, bronchial asthma or CHF

✣ lidocaine HCl

Trade: Lidocaine HCl, Lidopen Auto-Injector, Xylocaine HCl

Classification:

Antidysrhythmic (Class IB); local anesthetic

Action:

- Depresses phase O and suppresses ventricular arrhythmias by decreasing automaticity by reducing the slope of phase 4 diastolic depolarization

- Increases fibrillation threshold
- Cardiac depressant
- Terminates reentry ventricular dysrhythmias by reducing the ventricular refractory periods

Clinical Applications:

Used for the suppression of ventricular ectopy and ventricular tachycardia, for ventricular fibrillation, and for digitalis toxicity.

Dose:

Adult: 1-1.5 mg/kg body weight IV bolus over 1 min followed by a 0.5-0.75 mg/kg dose every 8 to 10 minutes, if needed, until a total of 3 mg/kg is given or ectopy suppressed, then drip (2 g/500 cc D_5W) at 1-4 mg/min or 20-50 µg/kg/min

Elderly: 0.5 mg/kg IV bolus, followed by 0.25 mg/kg dose q8-10 minutes, if needed until a total of 1.5 mg/kg is given or ectopy suppressed, then a drip at 20-50 µg/kg/min

Child: 1 mg/kg IV bolus, then drip (120 mg/100 cc D_5W) at 30 µg/kg/min [1-2.5 ml/kg/hr = 20-50 µg/kg/hr.]

Side Effects:

CNS: Confusion, convulsions, coma, dizziness, drowsiness, euphoria, headache, involuntary movements, paresthesias

CV: Bradycardia, cardiac arrest, heart block hypotension

GI: Anorexia, nausea, vomiting

EENT: Blurred vision, diplopia, tinnitus, slurred speech

INTEG: Edema, rash, urticaria

RESP: Dyspnea, respiratory depression

OTHER: Fever

Nursing Considerations:

Continuous cardiac monitoring must be used during administration. If ventricular ectopy increases, may need rebolus dose. Monitor blood levels of drug, especially in the elderly, and prn changes in neuro status (therapeutic 1.5-5.5 µg/ml). Notify MD of signs of toxicity. IV site should be monitored for infiltration as the patient may not feel discomfort due to anesthetic action of drug in tissues.

Precautions:

Use with caution in elderly, children, pregnancy (C), lactation, renal or liver disease, CHF, or malignant hyperthermia.

Contraindications:

Advanced AV block, Wolff-Parkinson-White Syndrome or hypersensitivity to amides. IV drip concentration of medicine should not be given IV push

✤ magnesium sulfate

Classification:

Anticonvulsant; magnesium replenisher

Action:

- Increases magnesium concentration to prevent dysrhythmias and coronary artery vasospasm that may be caused by magnesium deficiency
- Decreases acetylcholine in motor nerve terminals
- Decreases SA node impulse formation
- Magnesium replacement

Clinical Applications:

Used in the treatment of seizures caused by hypomagnesemia, pregnancy-induced hypertension, or acute nephritis. Experimentally, may be useful in acute MI to help prevent sudden death and with refractory torsades de pointes.

Dose:

MI

Adult: 4 cc of 50% solution (1 g/2 cc) [= 8 mmol MgSO4] diluted in enough sterile water to make 20 cc; IV push over 5 min, followed by IV drip (32 ml/250 cc D_5W) [= 65 mmol MgSO4] over 24 hrs

Seizures

Adult: 1-2 g IV over 15 min, then 1 g IM q4-6 hrs; maximum rate of 150 mg/min

Child: 20-40 mg/kg in 20% solution IM; repeat prn

Preeclampsia

Adult: 4 g/250 cc D5W IV and 4 g IM, then 4 g IM q4h prn; or 4 g IV loading dose, then 1-4 g IV/hr, not to exceed 3 cc/min or 150 mg/min; may be given as a single dose with 4 g/250 cc D5W IV over 3 hours

Side Effects:

CNS: Confusion, drowsiness, hypothermia, flaccid paralysis, decreased deep tendon reflexes, sedation, stupor

CV: Circulatory collapse, heart block, hypotension

GU: Polydipsia

INTEG; Flushing, sweating

RESP: Respiratory depression, paralysis

Nursing Considerations:

Cardiac monitoring should be used and is mandatory when given for MI. Notify MD of dysrhythmias or heart block. Assess VS: q15 min during IV administration; hold medication for respiratory rate less than 16/min. Assess I&O: notify MD for urinary output < 30 cc/hr. Assess reflexes for decrease (would signal magnesium toxicity) q1-2 hours. Monitor lab studies for magnesium levels. Calcium gluconate should be available for toxicity. Patient's room should be kept darkened, and stimuli should be decreased.

Precautions:

Use with caution in serious renal insufficiency or pregnancy (C). Incompatible with alkaline solutions.

Contraindications:

Hypersensitivity, renal disease, intestinal obstruction or perforation

✢ methyldopa

Trade: Aldomet, Amodopa, Methyldopa/Methyldopate HCl

Classification:

Antihypertensive

Action:

- Decreases CNS sympathetic outflow
- Decreases plasma renin activity
- Stimulates central inhibitory α-adrenergic receptors or acts as a false transmitter
- Decreases arterial pressure

Clinical Applications:

Used in the treatment of hypertension

Dose:

Adult: 250-500 mg/100 cc D5W IV q6h; run over 30-60 min; maximum of 1000 mg/6 hrs

250 mg PO bid or tid, then adjusted q2d as needed; 0.5-3 g PO qd in 2-4 divided doses for maintenance; maximum dose of 3 g/day

Child: 20-40 mg/kg/day IV in 4 divided doses; maximum of 65 mg/kg/day

10 mg/kg/day PO in 2-4 divided doses; maximum of 65 mg/kg/day or 3 g/day, whichever is least

Side Effects:

CNS: Depression, dizziness, drowsiness, headache, nightmares, involuntary movements, paresthesia, psychosis, sedation, weakness

CV: Angina, bradycardia, edema, myocarditis, orthostatic hypotension, weight gain

GI: Constipation, diarrhea, hepatic dysfunction or necrosis, nausea, vomiting

GU: Impotence, oliguria, polyuria

EENT: Dry mouth, nasal congestion, eczema, sore or black tongue

INTEG: Lupus-like syndrome, pruritus, rash

HEMA: Hemolytic anemia, positive Coombs' test, leukopenia, thrombocytopenia

Nursing Considerations:

Assess VS; observe for postural hypotension. Monitor lab studies for decreased platelet count, increased BUN and creatinine or changes in renal and liver function. Do not discontinue drug abruptly; taper over several days. Do not use over-the-counter cough, cold or allergy products unless approved by MD. Avoid exposure to sunlight or wear sunscreen. Urine may turn dark in toilet bowls cleaned with bleach.

Precautions:

Use with caution in pregnancy (C), eclampsia, or severe cardiac or liver disease.

Contraindications:

Active hepatic disease, blood dyscrasias, or hypersensitivity to sulfites

---

✣ metolazone

Trade: Diulo, Mykrox, Zaroxolyn

Classification:

Diuretic

Action:

- Increases urinary excretion of sodium, chloride, potassium, magnesium, and water
- Inhibits sodium reabsorption in the cortical diluting site of the ascending loop of Henle and proximal convoluted tubule

Clinical Applications:

Used in the treatment of hypertension and in the edema associated with CHF, renal disease, and furosemide-resistant edema

Dose:

Edema

Adult: 5-20 mg PO qd

Hypertension

Adult: 2.5-5 mg PO qd: maintenance dose determined by patient's B/P; Mykrox 0.5-1 mg PO qd

Side Effects:

CNS: Anxiety, depression, dizziness, drowsiness, fatigue, headache, paresthesia, syncope, weakness

CV: Chest pain, orthostatic hypotension, palpitations, irregular pulse, volume depletion

GI: Anorexia, constipation, cramps, diarrhea, GI irritation, hepatitis, nausea, pancreatitis, vomiting

GU: Azotemia, oliguria

EENT: Blurred vision

INTEG: Chills, fever, photosensitivity, purpura, rash, urticaria

HEMA: Aplastic anemia, hemolytic anemia, agranulocytosis, leukopenia, neutropenia, thrombocytopenia

ENDO: Increased BUN and creatinine, hypercalcemia, hyperglycemia, hyperuricemia, hypochloremia, hypokalemia, hypomagnesemia, hyponatremia

MS: Gout, joint pain, muscle cramps

Nursing Considerations:

Assess I&O; weigh daily. Drug effect may decrease with prolonged daily use. Maintain fluid balance. Observe mucous membranes and skin turgor for hydration. Observe for decrease in edema. Assess VS: dyspnea on exertion and postural hypotension may occur. Monitor lab studies for electrolyte imbalances, CBC and ABG changes, glucose in urine if the patient is a diabetic. Administer medication in morning to avoid nocturia.

Precautions:

Use with caution with hypokalemia, renal or hepatic disease, COPD, gout, lupus erythematosus, or diabetes. Be aware that Zaroxolyn and some other forms of drug are not equivalent in their actions.

Contraindications:

Hypersensitivity to thiazides or sulfonamides, with anuria, pregnancy (D), or lactation

---

✤ metoprolol

Trade: Lopressor, Betaloc

Classification:

Antihypertensive

Action:

- Cardioselective β-blocker
- β-1 blocker
- Inhibits β-2 receptors in bronchial and vascular muscles with higher doses
- Produces decreases in B/P, heart rate, and cardiac output
- Decreases elevated plasma renin levels
- Decreases rate of SA node and AV node conduction
- Decreases myocardial oxygen demand

Clinical Applications:
Used in mild to moderate hypertension, acute myocardial infarction, angina, and in long-term therapy to reduce mortality after MI.

Dose:

MI
Adult: 5 mg IV bolus over 1 min, every 2-5 min × 3 doses, then 50 mg PO 15 min after the last IV dose and q6h × 48 hrs; 100 mg PO bid maintenance for 3 months

Hypertension
Adult: 50 mg PO bid, or 100 mg PO qd: may give up to 200-450 mg PO in divided doses

Side Effects:

CNS: Anxiety, catatonia, confusion, depression, dizziness, fatigue, headache, hallucinations, insomnia, mental changes, nightmares, tiredness

CV: Bradycardia, CHF, second and third degree heart blocks, hypotension, peripheral vascular disease

GI: Dry mouth, diarrhea, ischemic colitis, flatulence, hiccoughs, nausea, vomiting, mesenteric arterial thrombosis

GU: Impotence, reduced libido

EENT: Blurred vision, dry burning eyes, sore throat, tinnitus

RESP: Increased airway resistance, bronchospasm, dyspnea, laryngospasm, wheezing

INTEG: Alopecia, cold extremities, fever, pruritus, rash

HEMA: Agranulocytosis, eosinophilia, purpura, thrombocytopenia

Nursing Considerations:

Continuous cardiac monitoring must be done with IV administration. Observe for any EKG changes. Assess VS: baseline B/P and pulse prior to initiation of therapy. Always check apical pulse before giving this drug and withhold for pulse less than 45/min and notify MD. If B/P is less than 90 mm Hg systolic, withhold drug and notify MD. Do not give this drug if patient is actively wheezing. Monitor I&O; weigh daily. Maintain fluid balance. Assess hydration status; skin turgor and mucous membranes. Observe for lower extremity edema. Monitor lab studies with baseline values for renal and liver functions. After IV administration, patient should remain supine for 3 hours. Do not discontinue drug abruptly after patient is on maintenance dose; taper gradually over 2 weeks. Do not take over-the-counter cold preparations or nasal decongestants without MD approval.

Precautions

Use with caution in pregnancy (C), lactation, diabetes, renal or thyroid disease, major surgery, COPD, heart failure, coronary artery disease, nonallergic bronchospasm or hepatic disease.

Contraindications:

Hypersensitivity to β-blockers, cardiogenic shock, advanced second and third degree heart block, bradycardia, CHF or bronchial asthma; incompatible with any drug in syringe or solution

✢ mexiletine HCl

Trade: Mexitil

Classification:

Antidysrhythmic (Class IB)

Action:

- Increases electrical stimulation threshold of ventricle, His-Purkinje suystem, which stabilizes cardiac membrane
- Inhibits sodium influx and reduces the rate of rise of phase O
- Decreases action potential duration

Clinical Applications:

Used for the treatment of life-threatening ventricular dysrhythmias and for unlabeled use with Wolff-Parkinson White (WPW) syndrome.

Dose:

Adult: 200-400 mg PO q8-12h; maximum dose is 1200 mg/day

Side Effects:

CNS: Change in sleep habits, confusion, depression, dizziness, fatigue, headache, short-term memory loss, nervousness, paresthesia, psychosis, seizures, speech difficulties, tremors, weakness

CV: Angina, AV block, arrest, bradycardia, cardiogenic shock, cardiovascular collapse, hypotension, palpitations, sinus node slowing, syncope, increasing ventricular dysrhythmias, left ventricular failure

GI: Abdominal pain, anorexia, altered taste, upper GI bleeding, diarrhea, dry mouth, hepatitis, hiccoughs, nausea, peptic ulcer, vomiting

GU: Urinary hesitancy, decreased libido

EENT: Blurred vision, hearing loss, tinnitus

INTEG: Alopecia, dry skin, rash, Stevens-Johnson syndrome

MS: Arthralgia, edema

RESP: Dyspnea, pneumonia, pulmonary embolism, pulmonary fibrosis

HEMA: Hypoplastic anemia, agranulocytosis, blood dyscrasias, leukopenia, SLE syndrome, thrombocytopenia

Nursing Considerations:

Continuous cardiac monitoring should be used. Observe for widening PR intervals or QRS intervals, and notify MD. Assess VS; observe for B/P changes, increased pulse or respiratory rate. Assess I&O; assess lung fields for crackles (rales). Monitor lab studies for electrolyte imbalances and drug levels.

Precautions:

Use with caution in pregnancy (C), lactation, children, renal or liver disease, CHF, respiratory depression, myasthenia gravis, pre-existing sinus node dysfunction, hypotension, or structural heart disease.

Contraindications:

Advanced second and third degree heart block without a pacemaker, cardiogenic shock, hypersensitivity to amides

✣ minoxidil

Trade: Loniten, Minodyl, Minoxidil, Rogaine

Classification:

Antihypertensive

Action:

- Relaxes arteriolar smooth muscle and causes peripheral vasodilation
- Decreases B/P, peripheral vascular resistance
- Increases renin secretion
- Increases heart rate
- Increases urinary output

Clinical Applications:

Used for severe hypertension not responsive to other therapeutics and topically for the treatment of alopecia.

Dose:

Hypertension

Adult: 5 mg PO qd; increase gradually up to a maximum of 100 mg/day; usual range is 10-40 mg PO qd.

Child <12 yr: 0.2 mg/kg/day; usual range 0.25-1 mg/kg/day; maximum dose of 50 mg/day

Alopecia

Adult: Apply to scalp, 1 cc of a 2% solution bid

Side Effects:

CNS: Depression, dizziness, drowsiness, fatigue, headache, sedation

CV: Angina, CHF, edema, severe rebound hypertension, peaked T wave, pericardial effusion, pulmonary edema, sodium and water retention, tachycardia, tamponade

GI: Nausea, vomiting

GU: Breast tenderness, gynecomastia

INTEG: Hirsutism, pruritus, rash, Stevens-Johnson syndrome

HEMA: Decreased hemoglobin, hematocrit, and erythrocyte count

Nursing Considerations:

Assess I&O; weigh daily. Notify MD for pitting edema, weight gain > 5 pounds per week or 2 pounds per day. Observe mucous membranes and skin turgor for hydration. Maintain fluid balance. Assess VS: observe for heart rate > 20 beats/min more than patient's normal, or for respiratory changes, and notify MD. Monitor lab studies for electrolyte imbalances and for renal and hepatic function.

Precautions:

Use with caution in pregnancy (C), lactation, children, elderly, renal disease, CHF, and coronary artery disease. Concurrent use of a diuretic and a β-blocker is recommended.

Contraindications:

Acute MI, dissecting aortic aneurysm, hypersensitivity, and pheochromocytoma

✤ moricizine

Trade: Ethmozine

Classification:

Antidysrhythmic, (Class I)

Action:

- Decreases the rate of phase O depolarization prolonging refractory period
- Shortens the action potential duration
- Depresses the inward influx when sodium mediates the effects
- Prolongs AV nodal and intraventricular conduction
- Shortens phase 2 and 3 repolarization

Clinical Applications:

Used for the treatment of symptomatic, life-threatening ventricular dysrhythmias.

Dose:

Adult: 10-15 mg/kg/day PO in 2-3 divided doses; usual dosage is 600-900 mg/day in 3 divided doses.

Side Effects:

CNS: Anxiety, asthenia, cerebrovascular episodes (TIAs), confusion, coma, depression, dizziness, euphoria, fatigue, headache, nervousness, perioral numbness, seizures, sleep disorders

CV: Bradycardia, cardiac arrest, chest pain, CHF, supraventricular dysrhythmias, dysrhythmias, hypertension, hypotension, MI, palpitations, thrombophlebitis

GI: Abdominal pain, diarrhea, nausea, vomiting

GU: Dysuria, incontinence, impotence, decreased libido, urinary retention

EENT: Diplopia, eye pain, nystagmus, periorbital edema, swelling of the lips and tongue, tinnitus

RESP: Apnea, asthma, cough, dyspnea, hyperventilation, pharyngitis, pulmonary embolism, sinusitis

MS: Musculoskeletal pain

INTEG: Fever

Nursing Considerations:

Cardiac monitoring should be used for initiating therapy. Notify MD for heart block or worsening dysrhythmias. Assess VS: monitor for B/P changes.

Assess I&O: observe for decrease in urinary output.
Assess lung fields for crackles (rales).

Precautions:

Use with caution in CHF, hypokalemia, hyperkalemia, sick sinus syndrome, pre-existing cardiac conduction problems, pregnancy (B), lactation, children, or impaired hepatic or renal function.

Contraindications:

Advanced second or third degree heart block; cardiogenic shock

---

✣ morphine sulfate

Trade: Morphine Sulfate, Roxanol, Roxanol 100, Roxanol Rescudose, Roxanol SR

Classification:

Narcotic analgesic

Action:

- Decreases pain impulse transmission by interacting with opioid receptors
- Produces both analgesic and hemodynamic effects
- Increases venous capacitance
- Decreases systemic vascular resistance
- Relieves pulmonary congestion
- Decreases myocardial oxygen requirements

Clinical Applications:

Used as the drug of choice for acute MI, for analgesia, and in the treatment of CHF/pulmonary edema.

Dose:

Adult: 2 to 5 mg IV over 1-2 min, every 5 minutes prn

4-15 mg IM, SQ q4h prn

10-30 mg PO q4h prn

Child: 0.1-0.2 mg/kg IV, IM, SQ, with maximum of 15 mg

Side Effects:

CNS: Confusion, dizziness, drowsiness, euphoria headache, sedation

CV: Bradycardia, B/P changes, palpitations

GI: Anorexia, constipation, cramps, nausea, vomiting

RESP: Respiratory depression

GU: Urinary retention

EENT: Blurred vision, diplopia, miosis, tinnitus

INTEG: Flushing, pruritus, rash

Nursing Considerations:

Assess VS for respiratory depression or significant B/P changes. Notify MD for respirations < 10/min. Assess for urinary retention. Administer antiemetic concurrently with medication to alleviate nausea or emesis.

Precautions:

Use cautiously with addictive personality, pregnancy (B), hepatic or renal disease, children younger than 18 years old, or in respiratory depression. Incompatible with bicarbonate solutions. Increases the effects of CNS depressants. Naloxone (Narcan) should be readily available for reversal [dose 0.2-0.8 mg IV over 1 min].

Contraindications:

Hypersensitivity, addiction, hemorrhage, increased intracranial pressure

✤ nadolol

Trade: Corgard

Classification:

Antihypertensive, antianginal

Action:

- Non-selective β-blocker
- Decreases B/P, heart rate, and cardiac output
- Slows the sinus rate and decreases AV node conduction
- Suppresses renin secretion
- Decreases myocardial oxygen demands
- Can increase LVEDP in heart failure

Clinical Applications:

Used for the treatment of chronic, stable angina and hypertension.

Dose:

Adult: 40 mg PO qd; increase by 40-80 mg q3-7 days; maintenance dose usually 40-240 mg/day for angina, 40-320 mg/day for hypertension

Side Effects:

CNS: Depression, disorientation, dizziness, fatigue, hallucinations, headache, lethargy, paresthesia, sedation

CV: AV block, bradycardias, chest pain, CHF, conduction disturbances, edema, hypotension, palpitations, peripheral vascular disease, vasodilation

GI: Colitis, constipation, cramps, diarrhea, dry mouth, flatulence, hepatomegaly, nausea, pancreatitis, taste distortion, vomiting

GU: Impotence, decreased libido

EENT: Dry mouth, eyes, and skin, sore throat, tinnitus, blurred vision

INTEG; Alopecia, fever, flushing, pruritus, rash

RESP: Increased airway resistance, bronchospasm, cough, dyspnea, laryngospasm, pharyngitis, respiratory dysfunction, wheezing

HEMA: Agranulocytosis, thrombocytopenia, elevated liver enzymes

Nursing Considerations:

Assess I&O: weigh daily and report gain of >2 pounds per day, > 5 pounds per week. Maintain fluid balance. Assess for lower extremity edema; monitor hydration with skin turgor and mucous membranes. Assess VS: a decrease in B/P may necessitate a corresponding decrease in dosage. Check apical pulse before giving this drug and if < 60/min, withhold dose and notify MD. Do not discontinue drug abruptly as it may precipitate angina or MI. Taper over 2 weeks. Do not use over-the-counter drugs unless MD approved. This drug may mask signs of shock and hypoglycemia.

Precautions:

Use with caution in pregnancy (C), lactation, diabetes, hyperthyroidism, peripheral vascular disease, myasthenia gravis, and renal disease

Contraindications:

Cardiac failure, cardiogenic shock, advanced heart block, bronchospastic disease, CHF, COPD, and bradycardia

✢ nitroglycerin

Trade: Nitro-Bid IV, Nitroglycerin, Tridil, Nitrostat, Nitro-Bid Plateau Caps, Nitrocine Timecaps, Nitroglyn, Nitrong, Nitro-Bid, Nitrol, Deponit, Minitran, Nitrodisc, Nitro-Dur, Nitrogard

Classification:

Vasodilatory coronary

Action:

- Relaxes vascular smooth muscle
- Relieves angina
- Increases coronary collateral blood flow
- Decreases left ventricular work load and wall tension
- Decreases preload and afterload
- Dilates large coronary arteries and peripheral arteries and veins

- Reduces systemic vascular resistance, pulmonary capillary wedge pressure, left ventricular end-diastolic pressure, and arterial pressure
- Decreases myocardial oxygen requirements
- Increases cardiac output
- Does not increase heart rate (if preload adequate)

Clinical Applications:

Used for the treatment of angina, hypertension, and congestive heart failure in patients with ischemic heart disease.

Dose:

Adult: 0.15 to 0.6 mg SL every 5 min prn, up to a maximum of 3 tablets in 15 min; may use 1 tab 5-15 min prior to activity for prophylaxis

0.4 mg/metered spray every 5 min prn, up to a maximum of 3 sprays/15 min

1-3 mg buccal tabs every 5 min prn, up to maximum of 3 tabs in 15 min

2.5 to 9 mg PO q6-8 hrs

1-4 inches applied topically q4-8 hrs; 1 extended release transdermal patch applied qd to an area free from hair

Drip with 50 mg in 250 cc D_5W or 0.9% NS, mix in glass bottle and use nonpolyvinyl chloride tubing without a filter. Begin titration at 5 µg/min, and increase by 5-10 µg/min every 3-5 min. If there is no significant response after 20 µg/min, increase by

170 Medications and Medication Tables

10-20 μg/min until desired response is achieved or systolic B/P < 90 mmHg.

Side Effects:

CNS: Dizziness, flushing, headache

CV: Collapse, hypotension, shock, syncope, tachycardia

GI: Nausea, vomiting

INTEG: Pallor, rash, sweating

RESP: Possible ventilation-perfusion mismatching

HEMA: Methemoglobinemia (at high doses)

Nursing Considerations:

Continuous cardiac monitoring with IV use. Monitor VS for B/P and heart rate changes. Hemodynamic monitoring is recommended. Assess for dizziness and headache, which may require a dosage change. If concentration of the solution is changed, flush tubing with new solution before connecting to patient.

Precautions:

Use with caution in postural hypotension, pregnancy (C) and lactation. IV use decreases therapeutic response of heparin; incompatible with any other solution or medication

Contraindications:

Severe anemia, hypovolemia, cerebral hemorrhage, and increased intracranial pressure

✤ nitroprusside sodium

Trade: Nitropress, Sodium Nitroprusside, Nipride

Classification:

Antihypertensive

Action:

- Directly relaxes effects of arterial and venous smooth muscle
- Decreases preload and afterload
- Decreases B/P
- Reduces peripheral arterial resistance
- Increases venous capacitance
- Increases cardiac output and stroke volume
- Reduces myocardial workload
- Reduces coronary perfusion to ischemic myocardium

Clinical Applications:

Used to treat hypertensive events (emergency), left ventricular failure, and to decrease bleeding by decreasing B/P in surgery.

Dose:

Adult: Drip (50 mg/250 cc D_5W), start at 0.5 µg/kg/min, and titrate for desired hemodynamic parameters; doses noted up to 10 µg/kg/min with average dose 3 µg/kg/min.

Side Effects:

CNS: Agitation, ataxia, coma, dizziness, headache, loss of consciousness, decreased reflexes, restlessness, twitching

CV: Distant heart sounds, palpitations

GI: Abdominal pain, nausea, vomiting

GU: Impotence

EENT: Blurred vision, tinnitus

META: Acidosis

INTEG: Irritation at IV site, pink color

RESP: Dyspnea, hypoxemia, rales

Nursing Considerations:

Continuous cardiac monitoring must be done. An arterial pressure line is recommended. Solution should be utilized within 24 hours if covered, and 4 hours if not covered. Assess VS; titrate medication based on B/P and/or hemodynamic parameters set by MD. Wrap infusion bottle/bag with light-resistant material (aluminum foil). Observe solution for color change and discard if highly discolored. (Normal color of solution has faint brownish tint). Check serum thiocyanate levels q1-3d. Observe for signs of thiocyanate toxicity: profound hypotension, metabolic acidosis, dyspnea, headache, loss of consciousness, ataxia, or vomiting; notify MD and discontinue drip.

Precautions:

Use with caution in pregnancy (C), children, electrolyte imbalances, renal or liver disease, hypothyroidism, elderly patients.

Contraindications:

Hypertension

✣ norepinephrine bitartrate

Trade: Levophed

Classification:

Adrenergic

Action:

- Naturally-occurring catecholamine
- Potent α-receptor agonist causing peripheral vasoconstriction, with minimal effect on β-receptors
- Increases myocardial contractility and heart rate
- Positive inotrope; dilates coronary arteries
- Increases systemic vascular resistance
- Increases B/P
- Increases myocardial oxygen demand and may decrease cardiac output

Clinical Applications:

Used for the treatment of hemodynamically significant hypotension refractory to other agents; used to treat cardiac arrest.

Dose:

Drip (4 mg/500 cc D5W or 0.9% NS); Start at 2 µg/min and titrate until systolic B/P is 90; usual dose is 2-12 µg/min

Side Effects:

CNS: Anxiety, dizziness, headache, insomnia, restlessness, tremors

CV: Angina, bradycardia, dysrhythmias, ectopy, hypertension, palpitations, tachycardia

GI: Nausea, vomiting

RESP: Dyspnea

GU: Decreased urine output

INTEG: Gangrene, tissue sloughing

Nursing Considerations:

Continuous cardiac monitoring must be used. Direct arterial monitoring pressure should be used. Decrease drug rate as B/P increases. Assess B/P and pulse q5-15 minutes during active titration. Strict I&O; notify MD for urine output of <30 cc/hr. If extravasation occurs, infiltrate area with phentolamine 5-10 mg with 10-15 cc NS. Run via central line when possible.

Precautions:

Hemodynamic monitoring recommended. Use with caution with arterial embolus, peripheral vascular disease, severe heart disease, hypertension, hyperthyroidism, or elderly patients; may cause hypertensive crisis with tricyclic antidepressants. Incompatible with alkaline solutions.

Contraindications:

Contraindicated in hypovolemia, (except as temporary measure), ventricular fibrillation, tachydysrhythmias, pregnancy (D), pheochromocytoma, peripheral or mesenteric thrombosis.

✣ penicillin g sodium

Trade: Crystapen

Classification:
Antibiotic

Action:

- Interferes with cell wall replication in bacterial organisms
- Alters osmotic pressure and causes cell death

Clinical Application:

Used for the treatment of empyema, gonorrhea, meningitis, osteomyelitis, gangrene, mastoiditis, pneumonia, tetanus, urinary tract infections, anthrax and prophylactically in rheumatic fever. Used for gram positive organisms (*S. aureus, S. pneumoniae, S. bovis, S. viridans, S. faecalis, S. pyogenes, B. anthracis, C. perfringens, C. tetani, C. diphtheriae, L. monocytogenes*), gram negative organisms (*N. gonorrhoeae, N. meningitides, Bacteroides, E. nucleatum, P. multocida, S. minor, S. moniliformis*), and for spirochetes (*T. pertenue, T. pallidum, B. recurrentis, L. icterohaemorrhagiae*).

Dose:

Infections

Adult: 12-30 million U/day IV/IM in divided doses q4h; mix according to package insert with at least 50 cc NS and give over 30 minutes-1 hour; may be given as a continuous infusion over 12-24 hrs.

Child: 25,000-300,000 U/day IV/IM in divided doses q4-12 hrs

Prophylaxis

Adult: 2 million U IV/IM 30 min-1 hr prior to procedure, then 1 million U 6 hrs after procedure

Side Effects:

CNS: Anxiety, convulsions, depression, hallucinations, lethargy

CV: Anaphylaxis, hypotension, respiratory difficulty

GI: Increased ALT or AST levels, abdominal pain, colitis, diarrhea, glossitis, nausea, vomiting

GU: Glomerulonephritis, hematuria, moniliasis, oliguria, proteinuria, vaginitis

HEMA: Anemia, increased bleeding time, bone marrow depression, granulocytopenia

META: Alkalosis, hyperkalemia, hypernatremia, hypokalemia

Nursing Considerations:

Assess VS; observe for changes in respiration, BP, or heart rate. Assess I&O; notify MD for hematuria or urine output < 30 cc/hr. Monitor lab studies for changes in renal or hepatic function.

Precautions:

Use with caution in pregnancy (B) or CHF caused by sodium content.

Contraindications:

Hypersensitivity to penicillins and in neonates

✤ phenytoin sodium

Trade: Dilantin, Dilantin Capsules, DiPhen, Diphenylan Sodium, Phenytoin oral suspension

Classification:

Anticonvulsant

Action:

- Inhibits spread of seizure activity in motor cortex
- Reduces the activity of the brain stem centers responsible for grand mal seizures
- Promotes sodium efflux from the neurons

Clinical Applications:

Used for the treatment of status epilepticus, nonepileptic seizures, generalized tonic-clonic seizures, ventricular dysrhythmias, migraines, digitalis-induced dysrhythmias, tic douloureaux, and in refractory torsades de pointes.

Dose:

Seizures:

Adult: Loading dose of 10-15 mg/kg IV slowly at rate no faster than 50 mg/min; then maintenance dose of 100 mg PO or IV q6-8 hrs

Loading dose of 1 g PO divided into 3 doses, given at 2 hour intervals, then maintenance dose begun 24 hours later, 300 mg PO (extended release) qd or 100 mg PO tid

Child: Loading dose of 15-20 mg/kg IV slowly; rate no faster than at 1-3 mg/kg/min; then maintenance dose of 5-7 mg/kg/min

5 mg/kg/day PO in 2-3 divided doses: further dosage increases are given in response to lab studies and patient response with maximum dose of 300 mg PO daily.

Ventricular Dysrhythmias

Adult: Loading dose of 1 g PO divided over 24 hr; then 500 mg/day × 2 days; 250 mg IV given over 5 min, until dysrhythmias subside or until 1 g is given, or 100 mg IV q15 min until dysrhythmias subside or until 1 g is given

Child: 3-8 mg/kg or 250 mg/m^2/day PO as a single dose or divided in 2 doses; 3-8 mg/kg IV given over several min, or 250 mg/m^2/day as a single dose or divided in 2 doses

Side Effects:

CNS: Aggression, asterixis, ataxia, confusion, depression, dizziness, drowsiness, headache, paresthesia, slurred speech, suicidal tendencies, tremors

CV: Cardiovascular collapse, hypotension, periarteritis nodosa, ventricular fibrillation

GI: Anorexia, constipation, hepatitis, jaundice, nausea, vomiting, weight loss

GU: Albuminuria, nephritis

EENT: Diplopia, gingival hyperplasia, nystagmus, blurred vision

INTEG: Hirsutism, soft tissue inflammation, lupus erythematosus, rash, sloughing, Stevens-Johnson syndrome, toxic epidermal necrolysis

MS: Arthralgia

HEMA: Agranulocytosis, megaloblastic anemia, leukopenia, thrombocytopenia

Nursing Considerations:

Continuous cardiac monitoring for IV administration. Observe for changes in rhythm or widening complexes. Assess VS: q5-15 min during IV loading dose. Notify MD for systolic B/P < 90 mmHg. Do not administer through IV lines containing dextrose. Flush IV line with NS before and after each dose of medicine. Use special diluent provided with medication. Use an in-line micron filter. Assess site frequently for infiltration or extravasation. Use larger veins when possible. Monitor lab studies for therapeutic drug level. CBC with platelets should be done q2 weeks until stable, then q1 mo × 12, then q3 mo. Notify MD if neutrophils are < $1600/mm^3$. Do not discontinue drug abruptly without a change to another anticonvulsant. Urine may turn pink.

Precautions:
Use with caution in hepatic or renal disease or in the elderly. Do not give parenteral form via IV infusion for long-term therapy due to lack of solubility. Drug is incompatible with any other drug in solution or syringe.

Contraindications:
Contraindicated in hypersensitivity to hydantoin, SA or AV block, bradycardia, or Adams-Stokes syndrome.

✣ potassium

Trade: Effer-K, K-Lyte, K-Lyte DS, Klorvess, Tri-K, Twin-K, Cena-K, Gen-K, K-Tab, K-Dur, K-Lyte/Cl Kaon-Cl, Kaochlor, Kay Ciel, Klor, Klor-Con, Klortrix, Klorvess, Micro-K, Potachlor, Potage, Potasalan, Potassium Chloride, Slow-K, Kaylixir, Potassium Gluconate

Classification
Electrolyte

Action:
- Electrolyte replenisher
- Necessary for nerve impulse transmission
- Necessary for maintaining normal renal function

- Necessary for contraction of cardiac, skeletal and smooth muscles

Clinical Application:

Used for the treatment of hypokalemia, digitalis intoxication, and prophylaxis for hypokalemia.

Dose:

Potassium Chloride

Adult: 40-100 mEq PO in divided doses tid or qid

20-60 mEq/L of IV fluid to run at rate no faster than 15 mEq/hr; should not exceed 150 mEq/day

Potassium Bicarbonate

Adult: 25-50 mEq dissolved in water 1-4 times daily

Potassium Acetate

Adult: 40-100 mEq PO/day in divided doses; for prophylaxis, 20 mEq/day in 2-4 divided doses

Child: Same as adult

Potassium Gluconate/Potassium Phosphate

Adult: 40-100 mEq/day in 3-4 divided doses

Side Effects:

CNS: Confusion, flaccid paralysis, paresthesias of extremities

CV: Arrest, bradycardias, cardiac depression, dysrhythmias, heart block, hypotension, widened QRS, prolonged PR, depressed ST, peaked T waves

GI: Abdominal pain, cramps, diarrhea, nausea, ulceration of small bowel, vomiting

GU: Oliguria

INTEG: Cold extremities, pallor, rash

Nursing Considerations:

Monitor EKG and hemodynamics if available. Monitor I&O; weigh daily. Notify MD for urine output < 30 cc/hr. Monitor lab studies for potassium levels and renal function. Use large lumen IV catheter and give slowly as a diluted solution. Observe for infusion site redness or pain. Observe for GI hemorrhage, pain, distention, nausea/vomiting or other bleeding. Dilute liquid forms in fluid with at least 4 ounces of fluid, preferably 8 ounces. Never give IV medication faster than 20 mEq/hr, and that should be done via a central line. Avoid scalp veins in children.

Precautions:

Use with caution in patients with heart disease and renal impairment, or with patients who use potassium-sparing diuretics.

Contraindications:

Addison's disease, hyperkalemia, acute dehydration, severe hemolytic disease, severe renal disease, or extensive tissue breakdown or injury.

✣ prazosin HCl

Trade: Minipress, Prazosin

Classification:

Antihypertensive

Action:

- Relaxes arteriolar and venous smooth muscle
- Dilates peripheral blood vessels
- Decreases peripheral vascular resistance and B/P
- α-adrenergic blocker

Clinical Applications:

Used for the treatment of hypertension, refractory CHF, and Raynaud's vasospasm.

Dose:

Adult: 1 mg PO bid or tid; if needed, may increase to 20 mg PO qd in divided doses: usual range is 6-15 mg/day; maximum dose 20-40 mg/day. First dose should be given before bedtime to prevent syncope

Side Effects:

CNS: Anxiety, depression, dizziness, drowsiness, fatigue, headache, paresthesias, syncope, vertigo, weakness

CV: Edema, orthostatic hypotension, rebound hypertension, palpitations, tachycardia

GI: Abdominal pain, constipation, diarrhea, nausea, pancreatitis, vomiting

GU: Incontinence, impotence, priapism, urinary frequency

EENT: Blurred vision, dry mouth, epistaxis, red sclera, tinnitus

RESP: Dyspnea

Nursing Considerations:

Assess I&O; weigh daily. Maintain fluid balance. Observe mucous membranes and skin turgor for hydration status, Monitor edema. Assess VS; if initial dose is > 1 mg, patient may develop a first-time syncopal episode. Observe for any respiratory distress or jugular vein distention. Monitor BUN and uric acid levels with long-term therapy.

Precautions:

Use with caution in pregnancy (C), children, and patients who are receiving other antihypertensive drugs. β-blockers and nitroglycerine used concurrently with this drug can cause increased hypotensive effects.

Contraindications:

Hypersensitivity

✜ procainamide HCl

Trade: Procan SR, Promine, Procainamide, Pronestyl, Sub-Quin, Rhythmin

Classification:

Antidysrhythmic (Class IA)

Action:

- Suppresses phase 4 diastolic depolarization
- Reduces the automaticity of ectopic pacemakers
- Slows intraventricular conduction for reducing the slope of phase 0 of the action potential
- Suppresses ventricular ectopy
- Increases the fibrillation threshold
- May terminate reentry ventricular arrhythmias
- May cause slight decrease in cardiac output

Clinical Applications:

Used for the suppression of ventricular premature beats, recurrent ventricular tachycardia that is not responsive to lidocaine, and for conversion of supraventricular dysrhythmias. Procainamide HCl is the drug of choice for Wolff-Parkinson-White syndrome.

Dose:

Adult: 30 mg/min IV up to a maximum of 17 mg/kg, until arrhythmia suppressed, hypotension ensues, or QRS widened by 50% or more; Drip (2 g/500 cc D_5W) at 1-4 mg/min

1 g PO loading dose, with 250-750 mg PO q4-6h; 500-1250 mg (extended-release) PO q6-8h.

Side Effects:

CNS: Confusion, dizziness, headache, restlessness, weakness

CV: Arrest, cardiovascular collapse, heart block, hypotension, pericarditis

GI: Anorexia, diarrhea, nausea, vomiting

INTEG: Edema, pruritus, rash

HEMA: Agranulocytosis, hemolytic anemia, neutropenia, SLE, thrombocytopenia

RESP: Asthma

Nursing Considerations:

Continuous cardiac monitoring must be used with IV administration. Notify MD for prolonged PR interval or QT intervals. Observe for increase in ectopy—may need to rebolus. Lab studies for assessment of therapeutic response and to monitor electrolytes. CBC with white cell differential should be done q week × 3 months to assess for agranulocytosis. Assess VS and monitor for respiratory depression and changes in lung sounds.

Precautions:

Use with caution in congestive heart failure, left bundle branch block, pregnancy (C), lactation, children, hepatic or renal insufficiency, or respiratory depression.

Contraindications:

Myasthenia gravis, advanced second or third degree heart block, hyperkalemia, intraventricular conduction defects, torsades de pointes, or lupus erythematosus

✣ propafenone

Trade: Rythmol

Classification:

Antidysrhythmic (Class IC)

Action:

- Slows AV conduction
- β-blocking activity
- Reduces membrane responsiveness and spontaneous automaticity
- Prolongs the refractory period or the action potential duration
- Reduces the upstroke velocity of phase O
- Suppresses recurrence of ventricular tachycardia

Clinical Applications:

Used for the treatment of severe, life-threatening ventricular dysrhythmias.

Dose:

Adult: 150 mg PO q8h, allow a 3-4 day interval before increasing dose; maximum dose is 300 mg q8h

Side Effects:

CNS: Coma, confusion, dizziness, disturbing dreams, headache, paresthesia, syncope

CV: Angina, sinus arrest, atrial flutter, AV block, AV dissociation, CHF, dysrhythmias, intraventricular conduction delay, palpitations, sinus arrest, sick sinus syndrome, sudden death, torsades de pointes, ventricular tachycardia

GI: Anorexia, constipation, dry mouth, dyspepsia, flatulence, hepatitis, abnormal liver function studies, nausea, vomiting

EENT: Taste alterations, tinnitus, blurred vision

INTEG: Flushing, rash

RESP: Apnea, dyspnea

HEMA: Agranulocytosis, anemia, increased bleeding time, granulocytopenia, leukopenia, increased liver enzymes, thrombocytopenia

Nursing Considerations:

Cardiac monitoring should be used during initiation of therapy. Notify MD of widening complexes or AV block. Assess VS; notify MD for hypotension, increased heart rate over patient's normal, or increased respiratory rate. Assess I&O; notify MD for decrease in urinary output < 30 cc/hr. Assess lung fields for rales.

Precautions:

Use with caution in CHF, hypokalemia, hyperkalemia, recent MI, nonallergic bronchospasm, pregnancy (C), lactation, children, hepatic or renal disease, or elderly patients.

Contraindications:

Cardiogenic shock, bradycardia, hypotension, severe electrolyte imbalances and any cardiac conduction disorder

✣ propranolol

Trade: Inderal, Inderal LA, Inderal 10, Inderal 20, Inderal 40, Inderal 60, Inderal 80, Ipran, Propranolol HCl, Propranolol Intensol

Classification:

Antihypertensive

Action:

- Nonselective β-blocker with negative inotropic and chronotropic properties
- Decreases cardiac contractility, heart rate, and cardiac output
- Limits renin release by kidneys
- May increase or decrease myocardial oxygen demand
- Has antiarrhythmic anesthetic type effects on membranes and has antimigraine effects

Clinical Applications:

Used for the treatment of chronic angina, hypertension, supraventricular dysrhythmias, some ventricular dysrhythmias, prophylaxis of migraines, essential tremors, idiopathic hypertropic subaortic stenosis (IHSS). Used to manage tachycardias of pheochromocytoma.

Dose:

Dysrhythmias

Adult: 0.5-3 mg IV bolus at rate of 1 mg/min; may repeat in 2-5 minutes prn; may dilute drug in 50 cc NaCl and infuse 1 mg over 10-15 min

10-30 mg PO tid or qid

Hypertension

Adult: 40 mg PO bid initially, increase up to 120-240 mg/day, bid or tid; 80 mg (extended release) PO qd initially; increase up to 120-180 mg (extended release) PO qd.

Angina

Adult: 80-320 mg PO bid, tid or qid; 80 mg (extended release) PO qd; usual dosage with extended release is 160 mg/day

MI

Adult: 180-240 mg/day in divided doses, 3-4 times per day

Pheochromocytoma

Adult: 60 mg PO qd × 3 days preoperatively, in divided doses, or 30 mg/day in divided doses for inoperable tumor

Migraine

Adult: 80 mg (extended release) PO qd; 80 mg PO qd in divided doses; may increase to 160-240 mg/day in divided doses

Tremors

Adult: 40 mg PO bid: usual dose is 120 mg/day

Side Effects:

CNS: Bizarre dreams, depression, disorientation, dizziness, fatigue, hallucinations, lethargy, paresthesia, weakness

CV: AV block, bradycardia, CHF, hypotension, peripheral vascular insufficiency, vasodilation

GI: Colitis, constipation, cramps, diarrhea, dry mouth, gastric pain, hepatomegaly, nausea, pancreatitis, vomiting

GU: Impotence, decreased libido, urinary tract infection

EENT: Blurred vision, dry eyes, laryngospasm, pharyngitis, sore throat

INTEG: Fever, pruritus, rash

MS: Arthralgia, muscle cramps, joint pain

HEMS: Agranulocytosis, thrombocytopenia

META: Hyperglycemia, hypoglycemia

OTHER: Facial swelling, weight change, Raynaud's phenomenon

RESP: Bronchospasm, dyspnea, laryngospasm

Nursing Considerations:

Continuous cardiac monitoring with IV administration. Observe for EKG changes. Assess I&O; weigh daily. Report gain of > 5 pounds per week or > 2 pounds per day. Maintain fluid balance. Observe skin turgor and mucous membranes for hydration status. Assess VS; B/P q5-10 minutes during IV administration. Monitor lab studies for hepatic enzyme changes. Do not take over-the-counter drugs unless MD approved. Do not discontinue drug abruptly; taper over 2 weeks to prevent cardiac damage.

Precautions:

Use with caution in pregnancy (C), diabetes, renal or hepatic disease, hyperthyroidism, children, myasthenia gravis, peripheral vascular disease, hypotension, CHF, or patients who are currently taking other antihypertensive medications.

Contraindications:

Hypersensitivity to the drug, cardiac failure secondary to pulmonary hypertension, advanced second or third degree heart block, asthma, bronchospastic disease, bradycardia, CHF, and cardiogenic shock

✜ quinidine

Trade: Quinalan, Cardioquin, Quinidine Sulfate, Cin-Quin, Quinadine gluconate

Classification:

Antidysrhythmic (Class IA)

Action:

- Prolongs conduction and the effective refractory period
- Slows heart rate and prevents atrial and ventricular aberrant rhythms
- Decreases myocardial excitability

Clinical Application

Used for the treatment of premature atrial and ventricular contractions, paroxysmal atrial tachycardia, atrial flutter/fibrillation, and ventricular tachycardia.

Dose:

Atrial Fibrillation

Adult: 200 mg q2-3h PO × 5-8 doses; may increase qd until sinus rhythm is restored or toxic effects are exhibited. Maximum dose is 3-4 g/day after digitalization

Paroxysmal Supraventricular Tachycardia

Adult: 400-600 mg PO q2-3h

Other Dysrhythmias

Adult: 50-200 mg PO as a test dose, then 200-400 mg PO q4-6h; 300 mg PO (extended release) q12h.

(Quinidine gluconate) 600 mg IM then 400 mg IM q2h, after test dose. IV drip 800 mg in 40 ml D_5W run at 16 mg/min

Child: 2 mg/kg PO as a test dose; then 3-6 mg/kg q2-3 hours for 5 doses PO qd

Side Effects:

CNS: Anxiety, ataxia, confusion, dizziness, headache, involuntary movement, irritability, psychosis, syncope

CV: Arrest, bradycardia, cardiovascular collapse, hypotension, third degree heart block, prolongation of QT interval, ventricular dysrhythmias, ventricular tachycardia, ventricular fibrillation

GI: Abdominal pain, anorexia, diarrhea, hepatitis, nausea, vomiting

EENT: Hearing loss, mydriasis, photosensitivity, tinnitus, blurred vision, disturbed color vision

INTEG: Angioedema, fever, flushing, photosensitivity, rash, swelling, systemic lupus erythematosus

RESP: Dyspnea, respiratory depression or arrest

HEMA: Agranulocytosis, hemolytic anemia, blood dyscrasias, hypoprothrombinemia, increase in CPK-MM, shift to the left in WBC differential, thrombocytopenia

Nursing Considerations:

Cardiac monitoring should be used, especially with IV administration. Notify MD of widening intervals (PR, QRS, QT). Assess VS; monitor B/P for fluctuations and heart rate for increase. Monitor lab studies for therapeutic levels (2-6 µg/ml). Periodic CBC, renal and liver profiles should be done, and medication discontinued for dysfunction or blood dyscrasias. Digoxin or verapamil should be given prior to starting Quinidine to avoid increases in ventricular rate.

Precautions:

Use with caution in pregnancy (C), lactation, children, renal or liver disease, potassium imbalance, CHF, or respiratory depression

Contraindications:

Conduction defects, third degree heart block, myasthenia gravis, or hypersensitivity to cinchona derivatives

✤ sodium bicarbonate

Trade: Sodium Bicarbonate

Classification:

Alkalinizer

Action:

- Short-acting systemic alkalizer
- Reverses acidosis

Clinical Applications:

Used in the treatment of metabolic acidosis, cardiac arrests with ventricular dysrhythmias, ventricular standstill, ventricular fibrillation, ventricular tachycardia of longer than 10 minutes duration and based on ABGs, and as a systemic and urinary alkalizer.

Dose:

Arrest

Adult: 1 mEq/kg IV bolus over 15-30 sec, followed by 0.5 mEq/kg every 10 minutes based on ABG values/situation

Child. Same as adult

Infant: 1 mEq/kg IV bolus over 30 sec, to maximum of 8 mEq/kg/day based on ABGs/situation

Acidosis

Adult: Drip (500 mEq /500 cc D$_5$W or 0.9% NS) at 2-5 mEq/kg over 4-8 hrs depending on ABGs, or lab CO$_2$, or pH; maximum 50 mEq/hr.

Child: Same as adult

Alkalinizer

Adult: 325-2000 mg PO qid

Child: 12-120 mg/kg/day PO

Side Effects:

CNS: Confusion, convulsions, headache, hyperreflexia, irritability, tetany, tremors, weakness

CV: Arrest, edema, irregular pulse

GI: Belching, distention, flatulence, paralytic ileus

GU: Renal calculi

RESP: Apnea, cyanosis, shallow respirations

META: Alkalosis

Nursing Considerations:

Obtain ABGs often during emergency situations. Assess I&O; weigh daily. Assess for edema or fluid overload.

Precautions:

Do not mix with catecholamines or other solutions.
Use with caution in pregnancy (C), toxemia, CHF, renal disease or cirrhosis.

Contraindications:

Hypocalcemia, peptic ulcer disease, or hypertension

✤ spironolactone

Trade: Aldactone, Alatone, Novospiroton, Sincomen

Classification:

Potassium-sparing diuretic

Action:

- Antagonizes aldosterone in the distal tubules
- Increases excretion of sodium and water with potassium and retention
- Decreases B/P

Clinical Applications:

Used in the treatment of hypertension—primary and secondary—hyperaldosteronism, and edema associated with cirrhosis and ascites, nephrotic syndrome, and CHF.

Dose:

Edema/hypertension

Adult: 25-200 mg PO qd in single or divided doses

Child: 3.3 mg/kg/day PO in single or divided doses

Hyperaldosteronism

Adult: 400 mg PO qd × 4 days or 3-4 weeks, depending on test; then maintenance dose of 100-400 mg PO qd

Side Effects:

CNS: Ataxia, confusion, drowsiness, headache

CV: Dysrhythmias

GI: Bleeding, cramps, diarrhea, gastritis, vomiting

GU: Amenorrhea, postmenopausal bleeding, deepening voice, gynecomastia, hirsutism, impotence, irregular menses

INTEG: Pruritus, rash

EENT: Dry mouth, thirst

HEMA: Decreased platelets and WBCs

ENDO: Hyperchloremic metabolic acidosis, hyperkalemia, hyponatremia

Nursing Considerations:

Assess I&O; weigh daily. Maintain fluid balance. Observe mucous membranes and skin turgor for hydration status. Assess VS; EKGs periodically for patients on long-term therapy. Monitor lab studies for electrolyte imbalance, increasing BUN and creatinine, and changes in ABGs.

Precautions:

Use with caution in dehydration, lactation, or hepatic disease. Drug may increase digoxin half-life and cause digoxin toxicity.

Contraindications:

Anuria, renal disease, hyperkalemia, or pregnancy

✤ timolol maleate

Trade: Blocadren, Timolol

Classification:

Antihypertensive

Action:

- Non-selective β-blocker
- Competitively blocks stimulation of β-adrenergic receptor within vascular smooth muscle
- Decreases positive chronotropic/inotropic activity
- Decreases the rate of SA node discharge and increases recovery time
- Slows conduction of AV node
- Decreases B/P, heart rate, cardiac output, and myocardial oxygen consumption
- Decreases plasma renin
- At high doses inhibits β-2 receptors in the bronchial system and increases air resistance

Clinical Applications:

Used in the treatment of mild to moderate hypertension, tachydysrhythmias, prophylaxis of migraines, and the reduction of mortality and chance of reinfarction after MI

Dose:

Hypertension

Adult: 10 mg PO bid, or 20 mg PO qd; may increase by 10 mg q2-3d; maximum dose is 60 mg/day

MI

Adult: 10 mg PO bid

Side Effects:

CNS: Anxiety, dizziness, fatigue, hallucinations, headache, insomnia, paresthesia, syncope

CV: Bradycardia, chest pain, CHF, claudication, dysrhythmias, edema, hypotension

GI: Abdominal pain, ischemic colitis, diarrhea, nausea, mesenteric arterial thrombosis, vomiting

GU: Frequency, impotence

EENT: Dry burning eyes, sore throat, visual changes

INTEG: Alopecia, fever, pruritus, rash

RESP: Bronchospasm, cough, dyspnea, laryngospasm, rales

Nursing Considerations:

Assess I&O; weigh daily. Observe for changes in edema. Observe skin turgor and mucous membranes for hydration status. Maintain fluid balance. Assess VS: B/P frequently during initial therapy, and periodically during treatment. Monitor lab studies with baseline values for renal and liver function prior to beginning therapy. Do not discontinue drug abruptly; taper over 2 weeks. Do not use over-the-counter nasal decongestants or cold preparations unless MD approved.

Precautions:

Use with caution in major surgery, pregnancy (C), lactation, renal or thyroid disease, diabetes, COPD, coronary artery disease or nonallergic bronchospasm.

Contraindications:

Hypersensitivity to β-blocker, asthma, severe COPD, cardiogenic shock, advanced second or third degree heart block, bradycardia, CHF or cardiac failure

✜ ticarcillin disodium

Trade: Ticaripen, Ticar, Timentin (with clavulanate potassium)

Classification

Antibiotic

Action:

- Interferes with cell wall replication of bacterial organism
- Alters osmotic pressure to cause organism death

Clinical Application:

Used for the treatment of infections involving the soft tissues, urinary tract, respiratory tract and bacterial septicemia. Used for gram positive organisms (*S. aureus, S. pneumonlae, S. faecalis, C. perfringens, C. tetani*) and for gram negative organisms (*N. gonorrhoeae, Bacteroides, F. nucleatum, E. coli, Salmonella, P. mirabilis, M. morganii, P. rettgeri,*

Enterobacter, P. aeruginosa, Serratia, Peptococcus, Eubacterium).

Dose:

Adult: 12-24 g/day IV/IM in divided doses q3-6h; mix 1 g in at least 4 cc sterile H$_2$O for injection, then dilute further in at least 10 cc D$_5$W or NS and give over at least 5 minutes; may be diluted in 50-100 cc and given over 30 minutes-2 hrs; may be given as continuous infusion.

Child: 50-300 mg/kg/day IV/IM in divided doses q4-8h

Neonates: 75-100 mg/kg IV over 8-12 hrs.

Side Effects

CNS: Anxiety, coma, convulsions, depression, hallucinations, lethargy, twitching

GI: Increased ALT and AST levels, abdominal pain, colitis, diarrhea, glossitis, nausea, vomiting

GU: Glomerulonephritis, hematuria, moniliasis, oliguria, proteinuria, vaginitis

HEMA: Anemia, increased bleeding time, bone marrow depression, granulocytopenia

META: Hypokalemia

Nursing Considerations:

Assess VS; observe for respiratory difficulty, wheezing or tightness in the chest. Assess I&O; notify MD for hematuria or urine output < 30 cc/hr. Monitor lab studies for renal or hepatic dysfunction as well as changes in blood studies.

Precautions:

Use with caution in pregnancy (B) or with hypersensitivy to cephalosporins

Contraindications:

Hypersensitivity to penicillins

✤ tocainide HCl

Trade: Tonocard

Classification:

Antidysrhythmic (Class IB)

Action:

- Decreases sodium and potassium
- Decreases excitability of myocardial cells
- Increases pulmonary artery pressures and causes slight increase in peripheral vascular resistance and systemic vascular resistance

Clinical Applications:

Used for the treatment of life-threatening ventricular dysrhythmias, and prophylactically to prevent tachydysrhythmias after MI.

Dose:

Adult: 600 mg PO loading dose; then 400 mg q8h, usual dosage is 400-600 mg PO q8h

Side Effects:

CNS: Anxiety, confusion, dizziness, headache, irritability, involuntary movement, nervousness, paresthesia, psychosis, seizures, tremors

CV: Angina, arrest, bradycardia, cardiovascular collapse, CHF, chest pain, heart block, hypotension, palpitations, tachycardia, ventricular dysrhythmias, left ventricular failure

GI: Anorexia, diarrhea, hepatitis, jaundice, nausea, vomiting

EENT: Hearing loss, nystagmus, sore throat, tinnitus, blurred vision

INTEG: Chills, edema, fever, rash, swelling, mouth ulcers, urticaria

RESP: Cough, dyspnea, pulmonary fibrosis, respiratory depression, wheezing

HEMA: Agranulocytosis, hypoplastic anemia, bruising, blood dyscrasias, leukopenia, thrombocytopenia

Nursing Considerations:

Cardiac monitoring should be used for initiation and titration of drug. Notify MD of conduction disorders or AV block. Assess VS: observe for B/P fluctuations. Assess I&O: observe for decreasing urinary output or crackles (rales) in lung fields. Monitor lab studies for therapeutic drug level (4-10 µg/ml). CBC with differential should be done prior to administration of drug, q week × 3 mo, and frequently thereafter. Chest X-rays should be done for respiratory complaints to rule out pneumonia or pulmonary fibrosis. Do not use over-the-counter cold, cough or allergy medications unless MD approved.

Precautions:

Use with caution in pregnancy (C), lactation, children, renal or liver disease, respiratory depression, myasthenia gravis, blood dyscrasias, known heart failure, or hypokalemia.

Contraindications:

AV block without use of a pacemaker, or hypersensitivity to amide-type anesthetics.

✣ triamterene

Trade: Dyrenium

Classification:

Potassium-sparing diuretic

Action:

- Inhibits reabsorption of sodium and chloride in exchange for potassium in the distal tubules
- Increases potassium retention with diuresis

Clinical Applications:

Used in the treatment of edema associated with CHF, cirrhosis, hyperaldosteronism, nephrotic syndrome and steroid-induced edema.

Dose:

Adult: 100 mg PO bid; maximum 300 mg PO

Child: 2-4 mg/kg/day in divided doses

Side Effects:

CNS: Dizziness, headache, weakness

CV: Anaphylaxis, hypotension

GI: Diarrhea, dry mouth, jaundice, liver disease, nausea, vomiting

GU: Azotemia, increased BUN and creatinine, bluish discoloration of urine, interstitial nephritis, kidney stones

EENT: Dry mouth, sore throat

INTEG: Photosensitivity, rash

HEMA: Megaloblastic anemia, low folic acid levels, thrombocytopenia

META: Acidosis, dehydration, hyperkalemia, hypochloremia, hyponatremia

Nursing Considerations:

Assess I&O; weigh daily. Maintain fluid balance. Observe mucous membranes and skin turgor for hydration status. Monitor changes in edema. Monitor lab studies for electrolyte imbalances, decreases in liver or renal function, or changes in ABGs. Administer medication in the morning to avoid nocturia. Do not discontinue drug abruptly; taper over 2 weeks. Avoid prolonged exposure to the sun.

Precautions:

Use with caution in dehydration, hepatic or renal disease, CHF, history of gouty arthritis or diabetes mellitus.

Contraindications:

Anuria, severe renal or hepatic disease, hyperkalemia, pregnancy (D), lactation, or concurrent use with other potassium-sparing diuretics

✤ verapamil HCl

Trade: Calan, Calan SR, Isoptin, Isoptin SR, Verapamil HCL, Verelan

Classification:

Calcium-channel blocker

Action:

- Inhibits calcium influx across the cell membrane during depolarization
- Slow channel-blocking properties, especially in cardiac and vascular smooth muscle with antiarrhythmic effects
- Reduces afterload and myocardial contractility
- Decreases systemic vascular resistance
- Decreases myocardial oxygen consumption
- Negative inotropic effects
- Decreases SA/AV node conduction
- Increases AV refractory period and interrupts reentry at the AV node
- Coronary vasodilation

Clinical Applications:

Used for the treatment of paroxysmal supraventricular tachycardias that do not require cardioversion in chronic, but stable, angina, hypertension, and adenosine-resistant supraventricular tachydysrhythmias.

Dose:

Adult: 2.5-5 mg/kg IV bolus given over 1-2 minutes, repeat with 5-10 mg IV 15-30 minutes after the first dose if needed

80 mg PO tid or qid, increasing every week, if needed, to maximum of 480 mg/day; 120-240 mg PO (extended release) either qd or bid

Elderly: IV bolus to be given over 3-4 min

Child: 1-15 yr: 0.1-0.3 mg/kg IV bolus (maximum 10 mg) given over > 2 min, repeat dose in 30 min, if needed

Child: 0-1 yr: 0.1-0.2 mg/kg IV bolus given over > 2 min, repeat dose in 30 min if needed

Side Effects:

CNS: Anxiety, confusion, depression, dizziness, drowsiness, headache, insomnia, weakness

CV: AV block, bradycardia, CHF, edema, hypotension, palpitations, tachycardia, ventricular asystole

GI: Constipation, diarrhea, elevated liver function studies, nausea

GU: Nocturia, polyuria

Nursing Considerations:

Continuous cardiac monitoring during IV administration; observe for changes in PR interval, QRS duration, and QT interval. Assess VS, especially B/P.

Withhold medication for systolic B/P <90 and notify MD. Do not use over-the-counter drugs unless approved by MD.

Precautions:

Use with caution in patients with hypotension, CHF, pregnancy (C), lactation, children, renal or hepatic disease, or muscular dystrophy.

Contraindications:

Severe hypotension, LV dysfunction, cardiogenic shock, sick sinus syndrome, second or third degree heart block, SA node dysfunction, Wolff-Parkinson-White syndrome or with concurrent use of IV β-blockers

APRESOLINE DRIP CHART
(100 mg/250 cc D₅W)

mg/hr	cc/hr
0.4	1
0.8	2
1.2	3
1.6	4
2.0	5
2.4	6
2.8	7
3.2	8
3.6	9
4.0	10
4.8	12
5.6	14
6.4	16
7.2	18
8.0	20

TRIDIL TABLE

ml/hr	25 mg TRIDIL in 250 cc D$_5$W 100 μg/ml μg NTG/min	50 mg TRIDIL in 250 cc D$_5$W 200 μg/ml μg NTG/min
3	5	10
6	10	20
12	20	40
24	40	80

Pitressin Drip Chart
(100 Units/250 cc D$_5$W)
0.1 U/min = 15 cc/hr
0.2 U/min = 30 cc/hr
0.3 U/min = 45 cc/hr
0.4 U/min = 60 cc/hr

STARTING RATES FOR VASOACTIVE DRUGS
(based on a 70 kg person for approximate µg/kg/min)

Dopamine	(400 mg/250 cc) (1600 µg/cc)	13 cc/hr for 5 µg/kg/min
Dobutrex	(500 mg/250 cc) (2000 µg/cc)	11 cc/hr for 5 µg/kg/min
Tridil	(50 mg/250 cc) (200 µg/cc)	3 cc/hr for 10 mg/min 2 cc/hr for 0.1 µg/kg/min
Inocor	(500 mg/100 cc) (2500 µg/cc)	8 cc/hr for 5 µg/kg /min
Nipride	(50 mg/250 cc) (200 µg/cc)	10 cc/hr for 0.5 µg/kg/min

METHOD FOR RAPID CALCULATION OF IV DRIPS

1. Calculate how many μg or mg of the drug per each ml:

$$\frac{\text{mg of drug}}{\text{ml of solution}} = \frac{\text{mg of drug}}{1000 \text{ ml}} \times \frac{1000 \text{ μg}}{1 \text{ mg}} = \frac{\text{μg}}{\text{ml}}$$

Divide mg of drug 1000/ml by 1000 to obtain mg of drug/ml

Example:

$$\frac{800 \text{ mg}}{500 \text{ mg}} = \frac{1600 \text{ mg}}{1000 \text{ ml}} \times \frac{1000 \text{ μg}}{1 \text{ mg}} = \frac{1600 \text{ μg}}{1 \text{ ml}}$$

2. To calculate drip rates expressed in micrograms per kilogram per minute you must know the concentration of the solution, the weight of the patient in kilograms, and the number of ml/hr at which the drug is being infused.

$$\frac{(\text{μg/ml}) \times (\text{ml/hr})}{(60 \text{ min/hr})(\text{kg of body weight})} = \text{μg/kg/min}$$

Example:

$$\frac{1600 \text{ (μg/ml)} \times (10 \text{ cc/hr})}{(60 \text{ min/hr}) \times (70 \text{ kg})} = \frac{16,000 \text{ (μg/hr)}}{4200 \text{ min/kg/hr}} = 3.80 \text{ μg/kg/min}$$

3. To calculate the drip rate when given a desired dosage in micrograms/kg/min, the following formula is used:

$$\frac{(\text{prescribed dose in } \mu g/kg/min)\ (60\ ml/hr)\ (kg\ body\ weight)}{\mu g/ml\ of\ the\ solution} = ml/hr$$

Example:
The doctor asks for dobutrex at 5 μg/kg/min; the patient weighs 54 kg, and the pharmacy sends the solution with 1000 μg.

$$\frac{(5\ \mu g/kg/min)\ (60\ min/hr)\ (54 kg)l/hr}{1000\ \mu g/ml} = 16.2\ or\ 16\ ml/hr$$

From Carol Burns, Focus on Critical Care, Vol. 15, No. 4, pages 46-48; Mosby-Year Book. Reprinted by permission of the publisher.

INOCOR CHART 500 mg in 100 cc NS

Body Weight

Rate cc/hr	lb kg	88 40	99 45	110 50	121 55	132 60	143 65	154 70	165 75	176 80	187 85	198 90	209 95	220 100	231 105	242 110
5		5.2	4.6	4.2	3.8	3.5	3.2	3.0	2.8	2.6	2.4	2.3	2.2	2.1	2.0	1.9
6		6.2	5.6	5.0	4.5	4.2	3.8	3.6	3.3	3.1	2.9	2.8	2.6	2.5	2.4	2.3
7		7.3	6.5	5.8	5.3	4.9	4.5	4.2	3.9	3.6	3.4	3.2	3.1	2.9	2.8	2.6
8		8.3	7.4	6.7	6.1	5.6	5.1	4.8	4.4	4.2	3.9	3.7	3.5	3.3	3.2	3.0
9		9.4	8.3	7.5	6.8	6.2	5.8	5.4	5.0	4.7	4.4	4.2	3.9	3.8	3.6	3.4
10		10.4	9.3	8.3	7.6	6.9	6.4	6.0	5.6	5.2	4.9	4.6	4.4	4.2	4.0	3.8
15		15.6	13.9	12.5	11.4	10.4	9.6	8.9	8.3	7.8	7.4	6.9	6.6	6.2	6.0	5.7
20		20.8	18.5	16.7	15.2	13.9	12.8	11.9	11.1	10.4	9.8	9.3	8.8	8.3	7.9	7.6

Dosage in μg/kg/min

NIPRIDE CHART 50 mg in 250 cc D5W

Body Weight

Flow Rate cc/hr	Quantity of Nipride µg/min	lb kg	77 35	88 40	99 45	110 50	121 55	132 60	143 65	154 70	165 75	176 80	187 85	198 90	209 95	220 100	231 105	242 110
5	16.7		.48	.42	.37	.33	.30	.28	.26	.24	.22	.21	.20	.19	.18	.17	.16	.15
10	33.3		.95	.83	.74	.67	.61	.56	.51	.48	.44	.42	.39	.37	.35	.33	.32	.30
15	50		1.4	1.25	1.1	1.0	.91	.83	.77	.71	.67	.63	.59	.56	.53	.50	.48	.45

Dosage in µg/kg/min

NIPRIDE CHART 50 mg in 250 cc D5W

Flow Rate cc/hr	Quantity of Nipride µg/min	lb kg	77 35	88 40	99 45	110 50	121 55	132 60	143 65	154 70	165 75	176 80	187 85	198 90	209 95	220 100	231 105	242 110
										Body Weight								
20	67		1.9	1.7	1.5	1.3	1.2	1.1	1.0	.95	.89	.84	.79	.74	.70	.67	.64	.61
25	83		2.4	2.1	1.8	1.7	1.5	1.4	1.3	1.2	1.1	1.0	.98	.93	.88	.83	.79	.76
30	100		2.9	2.5	2.2	2.0	1.8	1.7	1.5	1.4	1.3	1.3	1.2	1.1	1.1	1.0	.95	.91

Dosage in µg/kg/min

NIPRIDE CHART 50 mg in 250 cc D5W

Flow Rate cc/hr	Quantity of Nipride µg/min	lb / kg	77/35	88/40	99/45	110/50	121/55	132/60	143/65	154/70	165/75	176/80	187/85	198/90	209/95	220/100	231/105	242/110
35	117		3.3	2.9	2.6	2.3	2.1	2.0	1.8	1.7	1.6	1.5	1.4	1.3	1.2	1.2	1.1	1.1
40	133		3.8	3.3	3.0	2.7	2.4	2.2	2.0	1.9	1.8	1.7	1.6	1.5	1.4	1.3	1.3	1.2
45	150		4.3	3.8	3.3	3.0	2.7	2.5	2.3	2.1	2.0	1.9	1.8	1.7	1.6	1.5	1.4	1.4
50	167		4.8	4.2	3.7	3.3	3.0	2.8	2.6	2.4	2.3	2.2	2.0	1.9	1.8	1.7	1.6	1.5
55	183		5.2	4.6	4.1	3.7	3.3	3.1	2.8	2.6	2.4	2.3	2.2	2.0	1.9	1.8	1.7	1.7
60	200		5.7	5.0	4.4	4.0	3.6	3.3	3.1	2.9	2.7	2.5	2.4	2.2	2.1	2.0	1.9	1.8

NIPRIDE CHART 50 mg in 250 cc D5W

Flow Rate cc/hr	Quantity of Nipride μg/min	lb kg	77 35	88 40	99 45	110 50	121 55	132 60	143 65	154 70	165 75	176 80	187 85	198 90	209 95	220 100	231 105	242 110
65	217		6.2	5.4	4.8	4.3	3.9	3.6	3.3	3.1	2.9	2.7	2.6	2.5	2.3	2.2	2.1	2.0
70	233		6.7	5.8	5.2	4.7	4.2	3.9	3.6	3.3	3.1	2.9	2.7	2.6	2.4	2.3	2.2	2.1
75	250		7.1	6.3	5.6	5.0	4.5	4.2	3.8	3.6	3.3	3.1	2.9	2.8	2.6	2.5	2.4	2.3
80	267		7.6	6.7	5.9	5.3	4.8	4.5	4.1	3.8	3.6	3.3	3.1	3.0	2.8	2.7	2.5	2.4
85	283		8.1	7.1	6.3	5.7	5.1	4.7	4.3	4.0	3.8	3.5	3.3	3.1	3.0	2.8	2.7	2.6
90	300		8.6	7.5	6.7	6.0	5.5	5.0	4.6	4.3	4.0	3.8	3.5	3.3	3.2	3.0	2.9	2.7

Body Weight

Dosage in μg/kg/min

NIPRIDE CHART 50 mg in 250 cc D5W

Flow Rate cc/hr	Quantity of Nipride μg/min	lb kg	77 35	88 40	99 45	110 50	121 55	132 60	143 65	154 70	165 75	176 80	187 85	198 90	209 95	220 100	231 105	242 110
											Body Weight							
95	317		9.1	7.9	7.0	6.3	5.8	5.3	4.9	4.5	4.2	4.0	3.7	3.5	3.3	3.2	3.0	2.9
100	333		9.5	8.3	7.4	6.7	6.1	5.6	5.1	4.8	4.4	4.2	3.9	3.7	3.5	3.3	3.2	3.0

Dosage in μg/kg/min

DOBUTAMINE CHART 500 mg in 250 cc D5W

Flow Rate cc/hr	Quantity Dobutrex µg/min	lb kg	77 35	88 40	99 45	110 50	121 55	132 60	143 65	154 70	165 75	176 80	187 85	198 90	209 95
						Body Weight									
2	66.7		1.9	1.7	1.5	1.3	1.2	1.1	1.0	1.0	.88	.83	.78	.74	.70
3	100.0		2.9	2.5	2.2	2.0	1.8	1.7	1.5	1.4	1.3	1.2	1.1	1.1	1.0
4	133.3		3.8	3.3	3.0	2.7	2.4	2.2	2.1	1.9	1.8	1.7	1.6	1.5	1.4
5	166.7		4.8	4.2	3.7	3.3	3.0	2.8	2.6	2.4	2.2	2.1	2.0	1.9	1.8
6	200.0		5.7	5.0	4.4	4.0	3.6	3.3	3.1	2.9	2.7	2.5	2.2	2.1	2.0
7	233.3		6.7	5.8	5.2	4.7	4.2	3.9	3.6	3.3	3.1	2.9	2.7	2.5	2.4
8	266.7		7.6	6.7	5.9	5.3	4.9	4.5	4.1	3.8	3.5	3.3	3.1	2.9	2.8
9	300.0		8.6	7.5	6.7	6.0	5.5	5.0	4.6	4.3	4.0	3.8	3.5	3.3	3.2
10	333.3		9.5	8.3	7.4	6.7	6.1	5.6	5.1	4.8	4.4	4.2	3.9	3.7	3.5
12	400.0		11.4	10.0	8.9	8.0	7.3	6.7	6.2	5.7	5.3	5.0	4.7	4.4	4.2

Dosage in µg/kg/min

DOBUTAMINE CHART 500 mg in 250 cc D5W

Body Weight

Flow Rate cc/hr	Quantity Dobutrex µg/min	lb / kg	77 / 35	88 / 40	99 / 45	110 / 50	121 / 55	132 / 60	143 / 65	154 / 70	165 / 75	176 / 80	187 / 85	198 / 90	209 / 95
14	466.7		13.3	11.7	10.4	9.3	8.5	7.8	7.2	6.7	6.2	5.8	5.5	5.2	4.9
16	533.3		15.2	13.3	11.9	10.7	9.7	8.9	8.2	7.6	7.1	6.7	6.2	5.8	5.5
18	600.0		17.1	15.0	13.3	12.0	10.9	10.0	9.2	8.6	8.0	7.5	7.1	6.7	6.3
20	666.6		19.1	16.7	14.8	13.3	12.1	11.1	10.3	9.5	8.9	8.3	7.8	7.4	7.0

Dosage in µg/kg/min

DOPAMINE CHART 400 mg in 250 cc D5W

Flow Rate cc/hr	Quantity Dopamine μg/min	lb / kg	77 / 35	88 / 40	99 / 45	110 / 50	121 / 55	132 / 60	143 / 65	154 / 70	165 / 75	176 / 80	187 / 85	198 / 90	209 / 95	220 / 100	231 / 105	242 / 110
5	133.3		3.8	3.4	2.9	2.6	2.4	2.2	2.0	1.9	1.8	1.6	1.55	1.5	1.4	1.3	1.25	1.2
10	266.6		7.6	6.7	5.9	5.3	4.9	4.5	4.1	3.8	3.6	3.3	3.1	3.0	2.8	2.7	2.5	2.4
15	400		11	10	8.9	8.0	7.3	6.6	6.1	5.7	5.3	5.0	4.7	4.4	4.2	4.0	3.8	3.6
20	533.3		15	13	12	11	9.7	8.9	8.2	7.6	7.1	6.7	6.3	5.9	5.6	5.3	5.1	4.95
25	666.6		19	17	15	13	12	11	10	9.5	8.9	8.4	7.8	7.4	7.0	6.6	6.3	6.0

Body Weight

Dosage in μg/kg/min

DOPAMINE CHART 400 mg in 250 cc D5W

Body Weight

Flow Rate cc/hr	Quantity Dopamine μg/min	lb kg	77 35	88 40	99 45	110 50	121 55	132 60	143 65	154 70	165 75	176 80	187 85	198 90	209 95	220 100	231 105	242 110
30	800		23	20	18	16	15	13	12	11	11	10	9.4	8.9	8.4	8.0	7.6	7.3
35	933.3		27	23	21	19	17	16	14	13	12	12	11	10	9.8	9.3	8.9	8.5
40	1066.6		31	27	24	21	19	18	16	15	14	13	13	12	11	11	10	9.7
45	1200		34	30	27	24	22	20	18	17	16	15	14	13	13	12	11	11
50	1333.3		38	33	30	27	24	22	21	19	18	17	16	15	14	13	13	12
55	1466.6		42	37	33	29	27	24	22	21	19	18	17	16	15	15	14	13
60	1600		46	40	36	32	29	27	25	23	21	20	19	18	17	16	15	15
65	1733.3		49	44	38	34	31	29	26	25	23	21	20	20	18	17	16	16
70	1866.6		53	47	42	37	34	31	29	27	25	23	22	21	20	19	18	17
75	2000		57	51	44	39	36	33	30	29	27	24	23	23	21	20	19	18

DOPAMINE CHART 400 mg in 250 cc D5W

Flow Rate cc/hr	Quantity Dopamine μg/min	lb / kg	77/35	88/40	99/45	110/50	121/55	132/60	143/65	154/70	165/75	176/80	187/85	198/90	209/95	220/100	231/105	242/110
80	2133.3		61	53	47	43	39	36	33	31	28	27	25	24	23	21	20	19
85	2266.6		65	57	50	44	41	37	34	32	31	27	26	25	24	22	21	20
90	2400		69	60	53	48	44	40	37	34	32	30	28	27	25	24	23	22
95	2533.3		72	64	55	50	46	42	38	36	34	30	29	29	27	25	24	23
100	2666.6		76	67	59	53	49	45	41	38	36	33	31	30	28	27	25	34

Body Weight

Dosage in μg/kg/min

CHILDREN'S DOPAMINE CHART (50 mg/250 cc)

Flow Rate cc/hr	Quantity Dopamine μg/min	lb kg	2.2 1	4.4 2	6.6 3	8.8 4	11 5	22 10	33 15	44 20	55 25	66 30	77 35	88 40
1	3.33		3.33	1.67	1.11	0.83	0.67	0.33	0.22	0.17	0.13	0.11	0.10	0.08
2	6.66		6.66	3.33	2.22	1.67	1.33	0.67	0.44	0.33	0.27	0.22	0.19	0.17
3	9.99		9.99	5.00	3.33	2.50	2.00	1.00	0.67	0.50	0.40	0.33	0.29	0.25
4	13.32		13.32	6.66	4.44	3.33	2.66	1.33	0.89	0.67	0.53	0.44	0.38	0.33
5	16.65		16.65	8.33	5.55	4.16	3.33	1.67	1.11	0.83	0.67	0.56	0.48	0.42
6	19.98		19.98	9.99	6.66	5.00	4.00	2.00	1.33	1.00	0.80	0.67	0.57	0.50
7	23.31		23.31	11.66	7.77	5.83	4.66	2.33	1.55	1.17	0.93	0.78	0.67	0.58
8	26.64		26.64	13.32	8.88	6.66	5.33	2.66	1.78	1.33	1.07	0.89	0.76	0.67
9	29.97		29.97	14.99	9.99	7.49	5.99	3.00	2.00	1.50	1.20	1.00	0.86	0.75
10	33.30		33.30	16.65	11.10	8.33	6.66	3.33	2.22	1.67	1.33	1.11	0.95	0.83

Dosage in μg/kg/min

CHILDREN'S DOBUTREX CHART (75 mg/250 cc)

Flow Rate cc/hr	Quantity Dobutrex µg/min	lb kg	2.2 1	4.4 2	6.6 3	8.8 4	11 5	22 10	33 15	44 20	55 25	66 30	77 35	88 40
1	5		5.00	2.50	1.67	1.25	1.00	0.5	0.33	0.25	0.20	0.17	0.14	0.13
2	10		10.00	5.00	3.33	2.50	2.00	1.00	0.67	0.50	0.40	0.33	0.29	0.25
3	15		15.00	7.50	5.00	3.75	3.00	1.50	1.00	0.75	0.60	0.50	0.43	0.38
4	20		20.00	10.0	6.67	5.00	4.00	2.00	1.33	1.00	0.80	0.67	0.57	0.50
5	25		25.00	12.50	8.33	6.25	5.00	2.50	1.67	1.25	1.00	0.83	0.71	0.63
6	30		30.00	15.00	10.00	7.50	6.00	3.00	2.00	1.50	1.20	1.00	0.86	0.75
7	35		35.00	17.50	11.67	9.75	7.00	3.50	2.33	1.75	1.40	1.17	1.00	0.88
8	40		40.00	20.00	13.33	10.00	8.00	4.00	2.67	2.00	1.60	1.33	1.14	1.00
9	45		45.00	22.50	15.00	11.25	9.00	4.50	3.00	2.25	1.80	1.50	1.29	1.13
10	50		50.00	25.00	16.66	12.50	10.00	5.00	3.33	2.50	2.00	1.67	1.43	1.25

Dosage in µg/kg/min

Medications and Medication Tables

CARDIOVASCULAR DRUGS

I. Classified on a cellular level
   A. **Electrophysiological properties (interference with action potential)**

   Phase 0: Rapid depolarization of the cell when sodium ions influx in and electrical impulse changes from negative to positive (QRS).

   Phase 1: Influx of sodium slows, potassium continues to move out of cells.

   Phase 2: Recovery phase = plateau phase; calcium moves in and the cell is partially repolarized (ST).

   Phase 3: Potassium moves out, calcium and sodium stops, repolarization occurs (T wave).

   Phase 4: Resting phase, cell repolarization completed; potassium returns and action potential ready to occur (isoelectric segment after T); requires sodium/potassium pump + ATP.

   B. **The Classes**

   Class I agents

   Class IA: Depression of phase 0 and prolonged action potential: blocks fast channel, lengthens AP duration, used for atrial and ventricular arrhythmias.

   Class IB: Slight depression of phase 0; reduces maximal rate of phase 0 depolarization, shortens AP duration in purkinje fibers, used in treatment of VT associated with QT prolongation (ie, torsades de pointes).

Class IC: Marked depression of phase O; potent depressors of AP depolarization, marked reduction in conduction velocity.

Class II:
Reduces sympathetic excitation and depresses phase 4 depolarization, beta blockers; blockade of adrenergic stimulation of the cardiac pacemaker potentials.

Class III:
Prolongs action potential duration and lengthens effective refractory period of the cardiac muscle.

Class IV:
Selectively blocks myocardial channels and depresses phase 4 depolarization and lengthens phases 1 and 2 of repolarization; the calcium channel blockers.

Medications and Medication Tables

ALGORITHMS

TABLE OF CONTENTS

Adult Emergency Cardiac Care Algorithm 233
Ventricular Fibrillation/Pulseless
Ventricular Tachycardia Algorithm 235
Pulseless Electrical Activity or
Electromechanical Dissociation Algorithm 238
Asystole Algorithm 240
Bradycardia Algorithm 242
Electrical Cardioversion Algorithm 244
Hemodynamic Algorithm 245
Acute MI/CP Algorithm 246
Hypotension, Shock, and Acute Pulmonary
Edema Algorithm 247
Tachycardia Algorithm 250

The ICU Quick Reference 233

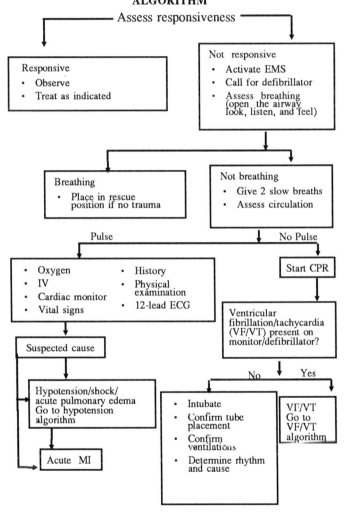

ADULT EMERGENCY CARDIAC CARE ALGORITHM

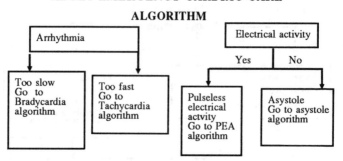

From JAMA, October 28, 1992, Vol 268, No. 16., pages 2216-2230. Copyright 1992, The American Medical Association. Used with permission.

VENTRICULAR FIBRILLATION/PULSELESS VENTRICULAR TACHYCARDIA ALGORITHM (VF/VT)

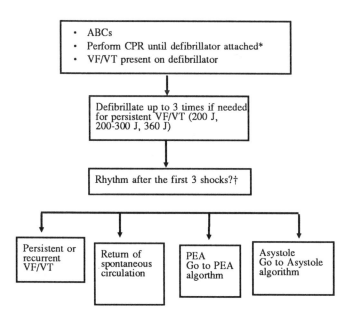

Algorithms

VENTRICULAR FIBRILLATION/PULSELESS VENTRICULAR TACHYCARDIA (VF/VT)

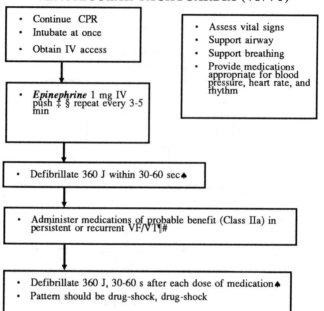

- Defibrillate 360 J within 30-60 sec♠

- Administer medications of probable benefit (Class IIa) in persistent or recurrent VF/VT¶#

- Defibrillate 360 J, 30-60 s after each dose of medication♠
- Pattern should be drug-shock, drug-shock

Class I: definitely helpful
Class IIa: acceptable, probably helpful
Class IIb: acceptable, possibly helpful
Class III: not indicated may be harmful
* Precordial thump is a Class IIb action in witnessed arrest, no pulse, and no defibrillator immediately available.
† Hypothermic cardiac arrest is treated differently after this point. See section on hypothemia.
‡ The recommended dose of *epinephrine* is 1 mg IV push every 3-5 min. if this approach fails, several Class IIb dosing regimens can be considered:

VENTRICULAR FIBRILLATION/PULSELESS VENTRICULAR TACHYCARDIA (VF/VT)

- Intermediate: *epinephrine* 2-5 mg IV push, every 3-5 min
- Escalating: *epinephrine* 1 mg-3 mg-5 mg IV push (3 min apart)
- High: *epinephrine* 0.1 mg/kg IV push, every 3-5 min
- § *Sodium bicarbonate* (1 mEq/kg) is Class I if patient has known preexisting hyperkalemia
- ♠ Multiple sequenced shocks (200 J, 200-300 J, 360 J) are acceptable here (Class I), especially when medications are delayed
- ¶*Lidocaine* 1.5 mg/kg IV push. Repeat in 3-5 min to total loading dose of 3 mg/kg: then use
- *Bretylium* 5 mg/kg IV Push. Repeat in 5 min at 10 mg/kg
- *Magnesium sulfate* 1-2 g IV in torsades de pointes or suspected hypomagnesemic state or severe refractory VF
- *Procainamide* 30 mg/min in refractory VF (maximum total of 17 mg/kg)
- #*Sodium bicarbonate* (1 mEq/kg IV):

Class IIa
  - If known preexisting bicarbonate-responsive acidosis
  - If overdose with tricyclic antidepressants
  - To alkalinize the urine in drug overdoses

Class IIb
  - If intubated and continued long arrest interval
  - Upon return of spontaneous circulation after long arrest interval

Class III
  - Hypoxic lactic acidosis

From JAMA, October 28, 1992, Vol 268, No. 16., pages 2216-2230. Copyright 1992, The American Medical Association. Used with permission.

PULSELESS ELECTRICAL ACTIVITY (PEA) OR ELECTROMECHANICAL DISSOCIATION (EMD) ALGORITHM

PEA includes:

- Electromechanical dissociation (EMD)
- Pseudo EMD
- Idioventricular rhythms
- Ventricular escape rhythms
- Bradyasystolic rhythms
- Postdefibrillation idioventricular rhythms

- Continue CPR
- Intubate at once

- Obtain IV access
- Assess blood flow using Doppler ultrasound

Consider possible causes
(Possible therapies and treatments)
- Hypovolemia (volume infusion)
- Hypoxia (ventilation)
- Cardiac tamponade (pericardiocentesis)
- Tension pneumothorax (needle decompression)
- Hypothermia (see hypothermia algorithm)
- Massive pulmonary embolism (surgery, thrombolytics)
- Drug overdoses such as tricyclics, digitalis, β-blockers, calcium channel blockers
- Hyperkalemia*
- Acidosis†
- Massive acute myocardial infarction

- *Epinephrine* 1 mg IV push,• ‡ repeat every 3-5 min

PULSELESS ELECTRICAL ACTIVITY (PEA) OR ELECTROMECHANICAL DISSOCIATION (EMD) ALGORITHM

↓

- If absolute bradycardia (< 60 beats/min) or relative bradycardia, give *atropine* 1 mg IV
- Repeat every 3-5 min up to a total of 0.04 mg/kg§

- Class I: definitely helpful
- Class IIa: acceptable, probably helpful
- Class IIb: acceptable, probably helpful
- Class III: not indicated, may be harmful

* *Sodium bicarbonate* 1 mEq/kg is Class I if patient has known preexisting hyperkalemia

†*Sodium bicarbonate* 1 mEq/kg:

Class IIa

- If known preexisting bicarbonate-responsive acidosis
- If overdose with tricyclic antidepressants
- To alkalinize the urine in drug overdoses

Class IIb

- If intubated and long arrest interval
- Upon return of spontaneous circulation after long arrest interval

Class III

- Hypoxic lactic acidosis

‡ The recommended dose of *epinephrine* is 1 mg IV push every 3-5 min

If this approach fails, several Class IIb dosing regimens can be considered.

- Intermediate: *epinephrine* is 2-5 mg IV push every 3-5 min
- Escalating: *epinephrine* 1 mg-3 mg-5mg IV push (3 min apart)
- High: *epinephrine* 0.1 mg/kg IV push, every 3-5 min

§ Shorter *atropine* dosing intervals are possibly helpful in cardiac arrest (Class IIb)

From JAMA, October 28, 1992, Vol 268, No. 16., pages 2216-2230. Copyright 1992, The American Medical Association. Used with permission.

ASYSTOLE ALGORITHM

- Continue CPR
- Intubate at once
- Obtain IV access
- Confirm asystole in more than one lead

↓

Consider possible causes
- Hypoxia
- Hyperkalemia
- Hypokalemia
- Preexisting acidosis
- Drug overdose
- Hypothermia

↓

Consider immediate transcutaneous pacing (TCP)*

↓

- *Epinephrine* 1 mg IV push, †‡ repeat every 3-5 min

↓

- *Atropine* 1 mg IV, repeat every 3-5 min up to a total of 0.04 mg/kg§♠

↓

Consider
- Termination of efforts¶

ASYSTOLE ALGORITHM

Class I: definitely helpful
Class IIa: acceptable, probably helpful
Class IIb: acceptable, possibly helpful
Class III: not indicated, may be harmful

* TCP is a Class IIb intervention. Lack of success may be due to delays in pacing. To be effective, TCP must be performed early, simultaneously with drugs. Evidence does not support routine use of TCP for asystole.

† The recommended dose *epinephrine* is 1 mg IV push every 3-5 min. If this approach fails, several Class IIb dosing regimens can be considered:
  - Intermediate: *epinephrine* 2-5 mg IV push, every 3-5 min
  - Escalating: *epinephrine* 1 mg-3 mg-5 mg IV push (3 min apart)
  - High *epinephrine* 0.1 mg/kg IV push, every 3-5 min

‡ *Sodium bicarbonate* 1 mEq/kg is Class I if patient has known preexisting hyperkalemia.

§ Shorter *atropine* dosing intervals are Class IIb in asystolic arrest.

♠ S*odium bicarbonate* 1 mEq/kg

Class IIIa
  - If known preexisting bicarbonate-responsive acidosis
  - If overdose with tricyclic antidepressants
  - To alkalinize the urine in drug overdoses
  - If intubated and continued long arrest interval
  - Upon return of spontaneous circulation after long arrest interval

Class III
  - Hypoxic lactic acidosis

¶ If patient remains in asystole or other agonal rhythms after successful intubation and initial medications and no reversible causes are identified, consider termination of resuscitative efforts by a physician. Consider interval since arrest

BRADYCARDIA ALGORITHM
(Patient not in cardiac arrest)

- Assess ABCs
- Secure airway
- Administer oxygen
- Start IV
- Attach monitor, pulse oximeter, and automatic sphygmomanometer
- Assess vital sign
- Review history
- Perform physical examination
- Order 12 lead ECG
- Order portable chest X-ray roentgenogram

Too slow (< 60 beats/min)

Bradycardia
Either absolute (< 60 beats/min) or relative

Serious signs or symptoms?*†

No

Type II second degree AV heart block? or third degree AV heart block? ♠

No → Observe

Yes → Prepare for transvenous pacer; Use TCP as a bridge device #

Yes

Intervention sequence
- *Atropine* 0.5-1.0 mg ‡§ (I & IIa)
- TCP, if available (I)
- *Dopamine* 5-20 µg/kg per min (IIb)
- *Epinephrine* 2-10 µg per min (IIb)
- *Isoproterenol* ¶

BRADYCARDIA ALGORITHM
(Patient not in cardiac arrest)

* Serious signs or symptoms must be related to the slow rate.

Clinical manifestations include:

Symptoms (chest pain, shortness of breath, decreased level of conciousness) and *signs* (low BP, shock, pulmonary congestion, CHF, acute MI).

† Do not delay TCP while awaiting IV access or for *atropine* to take effect if patient is symptomatic.

‡ Denervated transplanted hearts will not respond to *atropine*. Go at once to pacing, *catecholamine* infusion, or both.

§ *Atropine* should be given in repeat doses in 3-5 min up to total of 0.04 mg/kg. Consider shorter dosing intervals in severe clinical conditions.

It has been suggested that atropine should be used with caution in atrioventricular (AV) block at the His-Purkinje level (type II AV block and new third degree block with wide QRS complexes) (Class IIb)

♠ Never treat third-degree heart block plus ventricular escape beats with *lidocaine.*

¶ *Isoproterenol* should be used, if at all, with extreme caution. At low doses it is Class IIb (possibly helpful); at higher doses it is Class III (harmful)

\# Verify patient tolerance and mechanical capture. Use analgesia and sedation as needed.

From JAMA, October 28, 1992, Vol 268, No. 16., pages 2216-2230. Copyright 1992, The American Medical Association. Used with permission.

ELECTRICAL CARDIOVERSION ALGORITHM
(PATIENT NOT IN CARDIAC ARREST)

Tachycardia with serious signs and symptoms related to the tachycardia

↓

If ventricular rate is > 150 beats/min prepare for immediate cardioversion.
May give brief trial of medications based on specific arrhythmias. Immediate cardioversion is generally not needed for rates < 150 beats/min.

↓

Check
- Oxygen saturation
- Suction device
- IV line
- Intubation equipment

↓

Premedicate whenever possible*

↓

Synchronized cardioversion‡†
VT§
PSVT♠
Atrial fibrillation ⎯⎯⎯ 100 J, 200 J, 300 J, 360 J‡
Atrial flutter ♠

* Effective regimens have included a sedative (*eg. diazepam, midazolam, barbiturates, etomidate, ketamine, methohexital*) with or without an analgesic agent (*eg fentanyl, morphine, meperidine*). Many experts recommend anesthesia if service is readily available.

† Note possible need to resynchronize after each cardioversion.

‡ If delays in synchronization occur and clinical conditions are critical, go to immediate unsynchronized shocks.

§ Treat polymorphic VT (irregular form and rate) like VF: 200 J, 200-300 J, 360 J.

♠ PSVT and atrial flutter often respond to lower energy levels (start with 50 J)

HEMODYNAMIC ALGORITHM

	HIGH	LOW

AFTERLOAD (PVR OR SVR)	Dilators
	  Nipride
	  Nitrogylcerin
	  Nitrates
	  Inocor
	IABP
	  1:1 ratio
		Pressor Agents
		  Epinephrine
		  Norepinephrine
		  Dopamine
		  Neosynephrine
		IABP
		  1:1:3 1:4 ratio

PRELOAD (PCWP OR CVP)	Dilators
	  Nitroglycerin
	  Nitrates
	  Nipride
	  Inocor
	Diuretics
	  Lasix
	  Bumex
	  Edecrine
	  Mannitol
		Volume Agents
		  Colloids
		  Crystalloids
		  Blood
		  Hetastarch
		Anti-dysrhythmics
		  Lidocaine
		  Pronestyl
		  Bretylium
		  Pacemakers

Contractility (SVI or LVSWI)	β-blockers
	  Inderal
		Positive Inotropes
		  Dobutrex
		  Dopamine
		  Inocor

From JAMA, October 28, 1992, Vol 268, No. 16., pages 2216-2230. Copyright 1992, The American Medical Association. Used with permission.

ACUTE MI/CP ALGORITHM

Emergency Department
"Door-to-drug" team protocol approach
- Rapid triage of patients with chest pain
- Clinical decision maker established (emergency physician, cardiologist, or other)

ASSESSMENT

Immediate
- Vital signs with automatic B/P
- Oxygen saturation
- Start IV
- 12 lead ECG (MD review)
- Brief targeted history and physical
- Decide on eligibility for *thrombolytic* therapy

Soon:
- Chest roentgenogram
- Blood studies (electrolytes, enzymes, coagulation studies)
- Consult as needed

Treatments to consider if there is no evidence of coronary thrombosis plus no reason for exclusion (some but not all may be appropriate):

- *Oxygen* at 4 L/min
- *Nitroglycerin* SL, paste, or spray (if systolic blood pressure (>90 mm Hg)
- *Morphine* IV
- *Aspirin* PO
- *Thrombolytic* agents
- *Nitroglycerin* IV (limit systolic B/P drop to 10% if normotensive; 30% drop if hypertensive; never drop below 90 mm Hg systolic
- *β-blockers* IV
- *Heparin* IV
- Percutaneous transluminal coronary angioplasty
- Routine *lidocaine* administration is not recommended for all patients with AMI

From JAMA, October 28, 1992, Vol 268, No. 16., pages 2216-2230. Copyright 1992, The American Medical Association. Used with permission.

HYPOTENSION, SHOCK, AND ACUTE PULMONARY EDEMA ALGORITHM

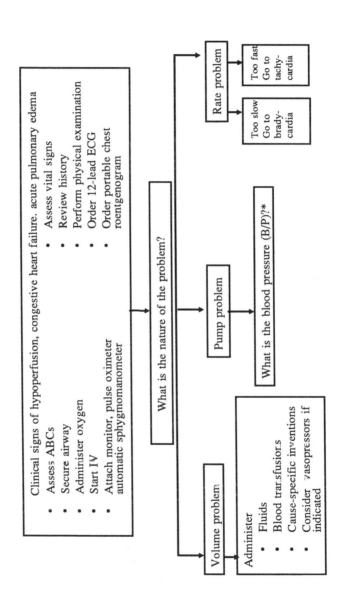

HYPOTENSION, SHOCK, AND ACUTE PULMONARY EDEMA ALGORITHM

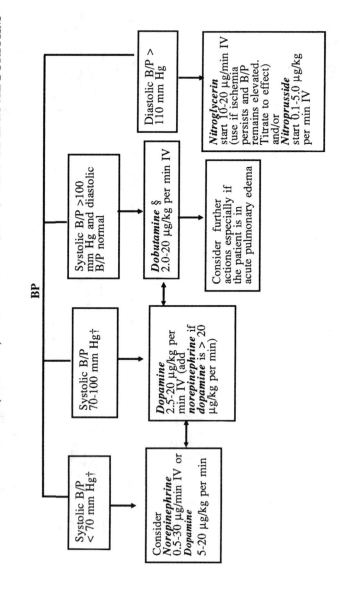

HYPOTENSION, SHOCK, AND ACUTE PULMONARY EDEMA ALGORITHM

First-line actions
- *Furosemide* IV 0.5-1.0 mg/kg
- *Morphine* IV 1-3 mg
- *Nitroglycerin* SL
- *Oxygen*/intubate PRN

Second-line actions
- *Nitroglycerin* IV (if B/P > 100 mm Hg)
- *Nitroprusside* IV (if B/P > 100 mm Hg)
- *Dopamine* (if B/P < 100 mm Hg)
- *Dobutamine* (if BP > 100 mm Hg)
- Positive end-expiratory pressure (PEEP)
- Continuous positive airway pressure (CPAP)

Third-line actions
- *Amrinone* 0.75 mg/kg then 5-15 µg/kg per min (if other drugs fail)
- *Aminophylline* 5 mg/kg (if wheezing)
- *Thrombolytic* therapy (if not in shock)
- *Digoxin* (if atrial fibrillation, supraventricular tachycardias)
- Angioplasty (if drugs fail)
- Intra-aortic balloon pump (bridge to surgery)
- Surgical interventions (valves, coronary artery bypass grafts, heart transplant)

* Base management after this point on invasive hemodynamic monitoring if possible.
† Fluid bolus of 250-500 mL normal saline should be tried. If no response, consider sympathomimetics.
‡ Move to *dopamine* and stop *norepinephrine* when B/P improves. Avoid *dobutamine* when systolic B/P < 100 mm Hg.
§ Add *dopamine* when B/P improves.

From *JAMA*, October 28, 1992, No. 16., pages 2216-2230. Copyright 1992, American Medical Association. Used with permission.

Algorithms

TACHYCARDIA ALGORITHM

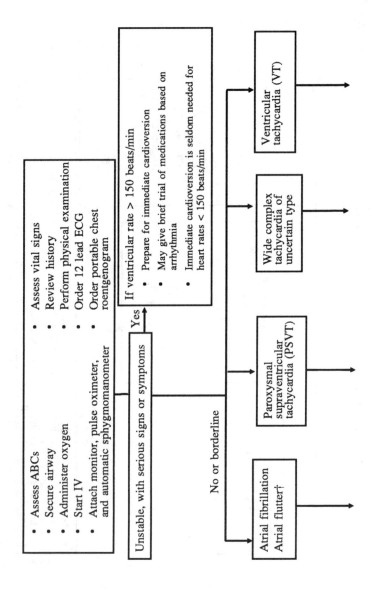

TACHYCARDIA ALGORITHM

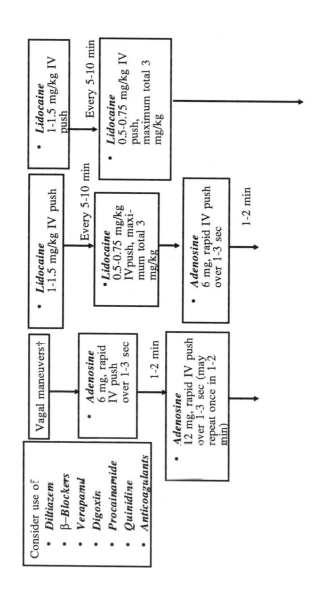

TACHYCARDIA ALGORITHM

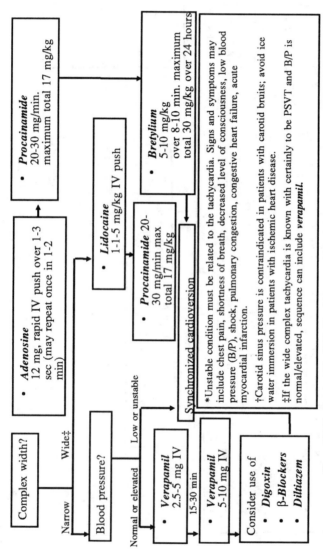

*Unstable condition must be related to the tachycardia. Signs and symptoms may include chest pain, shortness of breath, decreased level of consciousness, low blood pressure (B/P), shock, pulmonary congestion, congestive heart failure, acute myocardial infarction.

†Carotid sinus pressure is contraindicated in patients with carotid bruits; avoid ice water immersion in patients with ischemic heart disease.

‡If the wide complex tachycardia is known with certainly to be PSVT and B/P is normal/elevated, sequence can include *verapamil*.

From *JAMA, October 28, 1992, No. 16., pages 2216-2230. Copyright 1992, American Medical Association. Used with permission.*

HEMODYNAMIC MONITORING

TABLE OF CONTENTS

Preload	255
Afterload	256
Autonomic Nervous System	256
Formulas and Normals for Hemodynamic Parameters	258
Body Surface Area Chart	260
Fick Method of Computing Cardiac Output	261
PA Cathether Waveforms	264
Left Atrial Lines	268
Right Atrial Pressure Waveforms	265
Clinical Symptoms of Various Types of Shock States	267
Symptoms of Retroperitoneal Bleeding	269
Symptoms of Cardiac Tamponade	269
Comparing Shock's Three Stages	270
Continuous Mixed Venous Oxygen Saturation Monitoring	275
Pulmonary Artery Catheters	276
Troubleshooting a PA Monitor	279

PRELOAD

Related to volume and muscle stretch (measured by CVP [right side] or PCWP [left side])
   Factors affecting preload include:
- Increased mitral insufficiency
- Decreased mitral stenosis
- Increased volume
- Decreased volume
- Increased damage to LV affecting pumping ability
- Increased vasoconstrictors
- Decreased vasodilators
- Increased atrial kick
- Decreased intrathoracic pressure
- Decreased atrial natriuretic factor

Beth Minssen, R.N., M.S.N., C.C.R.N., Core Curriculum, Fourth Edition, 1990. Used by permission of the author.

AFTERLOAD

Resistance that must be overcome to propel blood forward (measured by PVR [right side] or SVR [left side]).

Factors affecting afterload
- Increased aortic stenosis
- Increased peripheral arterial vasoconstriction
- Increased hypertension
- Increased polycythemia
- Decreased intra-aortic balloon pump
- Increased vasoconstrictors
- Decreased vasodilators

Beth Minssen, R.N., M.S.N., C.C.R.N., Core Curriculum, Fourth Edition, 1990. Used by permission of the author.

AUTONOMIC NERVOUS SYSTEM
PARASYMPATHETIC

The parasympathetic fibers travel to SA node, atria and AV node. Parasympathetic control is responsible for the following functions:

- Decreased heart rate
- Decreased AV node conduction
- Decreased contractility (primarily atria)
- Decreased peristalsis of GI tract
- Changes in muscles for urination
- Constriction of pupils
- Gland secretion

SYMPATHETIC

Sympathetic fibers travel throughout the heart. Sympathetic control is responsible for the following functions:

- Increased heart rate
- Increased AV node conduction
- Increased contraction force (atria and ventricles)
- Increased metabolism
- Increased blood glucose
- Increased coagulation
- Vascular tone changes
- Bronchodilation
- Dilated pupils
- Decreased peristalsis of GI tract
- Increased adrenal cortical secretion

FORMULAS AND NORMALS FOR HEMODYNAMIC PARAMETERS

Body Surface Areas (BSA) Height and weight function Refer to Dubois chart	**Pulmonary Artery Pressure (PAP)** PAS = 20-30 mm Hg PAD = 8-15 mm Hg PAM = 15-20 mm Hg PCWP = 5-12 mm Hg or up to 14-16 mm Hg in compromised patients
Stroke Volume (SV) $SV = \dfrac{CO}{HR}$ 60-130 cc/beat or SV = LVEDV − LVESV	**Pulmonary Vascular Resistance (PVR)** $PVR = \dfrac{PAM - PCWP}{CO} \times 80$ 40-250 dynes/sec/cm^5
Stroke Volume Index (SVI) $SVI = \dfrac{SV}{BSA}$ or $SVI = \dfrac{CI}{HR}$ 35-50 cc/m^2/beat	**Pulmonary Vascular Resistance Index (PVRI)** $PVRI = \dfrac{PAM - PCWP}{CI} \times 80$ 255-285 dyne/sec/cm^5 − m^2
Cardiac Output (CO) [measured] CO = HR × SV 4-8 L/min	**Systemic Vascular Resistance (SVR)** $SVR = \dfrac{MAP - CVP}{CO} \times 80$ 800-1200 dynes/sec/cm^5
Cardiac Index (CI) $CI = \dfrac{CO}{BSA}$ 2.5-4 L/min/m^2	**Systemic Vascular Resistance Index (SVRI)** $SVRI = \dfrac{MAP - CVP}{CI} \times 80$ 1970-2390 dynes/sec/cm^5 − m^2

	Total Peripheral Resistance (TPR) $TPR = \dfrac{PAM}{CO}$ 2-5 mm Hg/L/min
Central Venous Pressure (CVP) [right atrial PA pressure] 2-6 mm Hg or 2-10 cm H$_2$O	Left Ventricular Stroke Work Index (LVSWI) LVSWI = (MAP− PCWP) × SVI × 0.0136 35-85 g/m/m^2/beat
Left Atrial Pressure (LAP) Mean 4-12 mm Hg	
Right Ventricular (RV) Pressure Systolic 20-30 mm Hg Diastolic 0-5 mm Hg End-diastolic 2-6 mm Hg Mean 2-6 mm Hg	
Mean Arterial Pressure (MAP) $MAP = \dfrac{SBP + (2 \times DBP)}{3}$ $MAP = \dfrac{(SBP - DBP)}{3} + DBP$ 70-90 mm Hg	Right Ventricular Stroke Work Index (RVSWI) RVSWI = (PAM − CVP) × SVI × 0.0136 7-12 g/m/m^2/beat
BSA = (weight in kg)$^{0.425}$ × (height in cm)$^{0.725}$ × 0.007184	
Ejection Fraction (EF) EF = $\dfrac{EDV - ESV}{EDV}$ 60-75 % of EDV	

BODY SURFACE AREA CHART

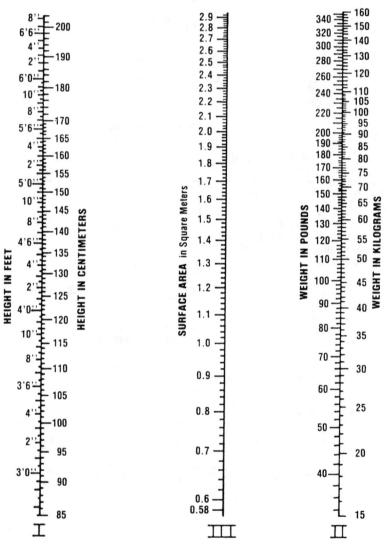

Place a straight edge across the chart so that height and weight are aligned. The body surface area is read on the center column.

FICK METHOD OF COMPUTING CARDIAC OUTPUT

The Fick method of determining cardiac output is based on the idea that the difference between arterial and mixed venous oxygen concentrations reflect the oxygen uptake as it flows through the lungs, and that oxygen removal from inspired air over a given time period reflects oxygen consumption. If the oxygen saturations of mixed venous blood and arterial blood are measured, the amount of blood flowing through the lungs can be calculated using this formula:

Cardiac output (CO) in:
$$\text{ml/min} = \frac{\text{Estimated oxygen consumption ml/min}}{\text{Arterial oxygen content} - \text{Venous oxygen content}}$$

or

$$CO = \frac{BSA \times 125}{CaO_2 - CvO_2}$$

or

$$CO = \frac{BSA \times 125}{(Hmg \times 1.34 \times SaO_2) - (Hmg \times 1.34 \times SvO_2)} \times 100$$

CaO_2 = Arterial oxygen content =
Hemoglobin (G/100 ml) × 1.34 × arterial oxygen saturation

CvO_2 = Venous oxygen content =
Hemoglobin × 1.34 × mixed venous oxygen saturation (SaO_2)

Estimated oxygen consumption = Body surface area × 125

Hemodynamic Monitoring

What is the cardiac output of a man who has a BSA of 1.5 m^2, a hemoglobin of 14.5, an arterial oxygen saturation of 95%, and a mixed venous oxygen saturation of 74%?

$$CO = \frac{1.5 \times 125}{(14.5 \times 1.34 \times 0.95) - (14.5 \times 1.34 \times 0.74)} \times 100$$

$$CO = \frac{187.5}{18.46 - 14.38} \times 100$$

$$CO = \frac{187.5}{4.08} \times 100$$

$$CO = 45.9 \times 100$$

$$CO = 4595 \text{ ml/min}$$

Answer: CO = 4.60 L/min

PA CATHETER WAVEFORMS

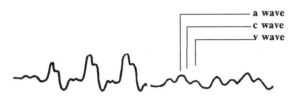

PAP waveform   PAWP waveform

a Wave: Corresponds to the EKG's P wave—the left atrium contracts.

c Wave: Corresponds to the closure of the tricuspid valve and may not be visible in the waveform because wave pressure is very low at this point.

v Wave: Corresponds to the EKG's T wave—the left ventricle contracts and the mitral valve bulges into the left atrium.

LEFT ATRIAL (LA) PRESSURE WAVEFORMS

a Wave Represents when the left atrium contracts and the mitral valve closes.

v Wave Represents when the left ventricle contracts and the mitral valve opens, and the left ventricle begins to fill with blood.

LEFT ATRIAL (LA) LINES

- Insert during CABG surgery, either via the pulmonary vein and guided into the left atrium or by a direct threading into the left atrium.
- It is extremely important that **ABSOLUTELY NO AIR** is introduced into line since this provides a direct route to the systemic and cerebral circulation; remove air from the fluid bag and use an in-line filter with the system.
- Aspirate, rather than flush through, any clots that might be noted in the line.
- Never give medications through the LA line.
- Never do the fast flush (or square waveform) calibration check with LA lines; line should be calibrated every eight hours and prn using the patient's phlebostatic axis.
- The patient should be either flat in bed or with the head of the bed elevated 20 degrees for consistency in readings.
- Simultaneous EKG and LA pressures should be recorded at least every 4-8 hours; LA pressures should be recorded every hour, including systolic, diastolic, and mean readings.
- Observe the line waveform for migration into the left ventricle; large **a** and **v waves** will be noted if this occurs.
- Dressing care must be done using sterile technique.

DISCONTINUING THE LA LINE

- Close all stopcocks to the patient.
- Remove sutures using sterile technique and pull the LA line out gently, followed by the application of a sterile dressing.
- Leave the mediastinal chest tube in at least 1-2 days following the LA line removal to observe for increases in bleeding and the possible complication of cardiac tamponade.

RIGHT ATRIAL (RA) PRESSURE WAVEFORMS

a Wave: Occurs when the pressure rises in atrial systole and the right atrium contracts; corresponds with the end of the PR interval or on the QRS on the EKG

x Descent: The slope of the **a wave**; occurs when the pressure decreases in the right atrium and the tricuspid valve closes

c Wave: Occurs during the closure of the tricuspid valve; the right ventricle begins to contract, right ventricular pressure increases, the pulmonic valve opens

v Wave: Occurs when blood is ejected into the pulmonary artery, the pressure rises during ventricular systole while the right atrium is filling with blood; corresponds to the T wave on the EKG

y Descent: The slope of the **v wave**; occurs when the tricuspid valve opens; the right ventricle begins to fill with blood from the right atrium

- In cardiac tamponade, the **x descent** is greater than the **y descent**.
- In tricuspid regurgitation, there will be a giant **v wave** and a large **y descent**.
- In mitral regurgitation, there will be a giant **v wave**, and the PCWP will not be an accurate indicator. Instead, use the mean of the **a wave**:

$$\overline{CVP} = \frac{\text{height of } \mathbf{a\ wave} + \text{height of } \mathbf{v\ wave}}{2}$$

CLINICAL SYMPTOMS OF VARIOUS TYPES OF SHOCK STATES

CARDIOGENIC SHOCK
- SBP less than 80 mm Hg
- Distended neck veins
- Elevated CVP
- Elevated PCWP (> 18)
- Elevated SVR
- Decreased CO/CI
- Pulmonary congestion
- Edema

HYPOVOLEMIC SHOCK
- Flat neck veins
- Decreased CVP
- Decreased PA pressure
- Decreased CO/CI
- Decreased PCWP

SEPTIC SHOCK (WARM PHASE)
- Chills
- Hyperthermia
- Hypoxemia
- ARDS
- Pulmonary edema
- Decreased SVR
- Increased heart rate
- Increased respirations
- Decreased urine output
- Warm, flushed skin

- Confusion, restlessness fatigue
- Initial increase or normal CO
- Decreased MABP (< 60 mm Hg)

SEPTIC SHOCK (COLD PHASE)
- Decreased CO/CI
- Elevated SVR
- Severe hypotension
- Increased tachycardia
- Hypothermia
- Cold and clammy skin
- Peripheral pulses are weak and thready or absent
- Multiple system organ failure
- Coma and death

ANAPHYLACTIC SHOCK
- Hypotension
- Nausea, vomiting, diarrhea
- Wheezing
- Seizures
- Anxiety
- Warm, moist skin, pallor
- Urticaria
- Bronchospasm, laryngospasm
- Dysrhythmias
- Stridor
- Confusion
- Abdominal pain, cramping

NEUROGENIC SHOCK
- Decreased heart rate
- Decreased CO/CI
- Decreased SVR

- Hypotension
- Decreased urine output
- Increased respiratory rate
- Confusion, restlessness

SYMPTOMS OF RETROPERITONEAL BLEEDING

- Increased heart rate
- Decreased blood pressure
- Narrowing pulse pressure
- Cool, pale, clammy skin
- Decreased hemoglobin and hematocrit
- Grey Turner's sign

SYMPTOMS OF CARDIAC TAMPONADE

- Beck's Triad:
  - Decreased blood pressure (SBP less than 100 mm hg)
  - Muffled or diminished heart sounds
  - JVD with patient's head of bed elevated 30-45 degrees
- Increased venous pressure (increased CVP over 20)
- Dyspnea
- Kussmaul's sign
- Pulsus paradoxicus *(feel pulse and if it disappears on patient's inspiration, this is pulsus paradoxicus)*
- Cyanosis
- Decreased CO/CI

- Pulse rate increased 20 beats/min or more from normal SBP, decreased 20 mm Hg or more from normal
- Pulse pressure narrows
- Cardiac pressures equalize (RA, PAD, PCWP, LA)
- Electrical alternans

COMPARING SHOCK'S THREE STAGES
Parameter
  Level of consciousness
  (Alterations caused by hypoxia, hypocapnia, and sympathetic catecholamine release.)

Early Stage
- Restlessness
- Anxiety
- Impaired memory
- Agitation
- Confusion

Middle Stage
- Lethargy, weakness, fatigue
- Unresponsiveness
- Decreasing motor responses
- Inappropriate behavior

Late Stage
- Unresponsiveness
- Cerebral ischemia

Parameter
  Blood pressure

Early Stage
- Normal or adequate B/P to perfuse vital organs
- Increased stroke volume (can cause SBP to increase)
- Systemic arteriolar vasoconstriction (can cause DBP to decrease)

Middle Stage
- Normal to decreasing B/P
- Pulse pressure narrows
- SBP decreased from decreased stroke volume
- DBP increased from increased vasoconstriction
- Paradoxical pulse may occur

Late Stage
- Marked hypotension and widened pulse pressure, (caused by sympathetic tone loss)
- Cardiovascular collapse occurs

Parameter
  Pulse

Early Stage
- Possible sinus tachycardia

Middle Stage
- Sinus tachycardia continues, but various dysrhythmias may occur in addition

- Peripheral pulses become weak, rapid, and thready
- Blood flow is decreased to peripheral areas
- Pulse deteriorates as shock worsens
- Stroke volume decreases

Late Stage
- Extremely slow, and weak or absent pulse

Parameter

Respirations

Early Stage
- Rapid and deep (from respiratory alkalosis and reduced oxygenation)

Middle Stage
- Tachypnea continues
- Respirations may become shallow from hypoventilation
- Shortness of breath is experienced
- Crackles (rales), or wheezes are heard on auscultation
- Adult respiratory distress syndrome may occur

Late Stage
- Tachypnea or slow, shallow respirations

Parameter

Urine output

Early Stage
- Decreased urine output

Middle Stage
- Decrease in urine output worsens

Late Stage
- Severely decreased urine output
- Anuria
- Kidney failure

Parameter
  Skin

Early Stage
- Cool, pale, and clammy

Middle Stage
- Pale or cyanotic—possibly cold or clammy
- Nail beds may have decreased capillary refill
- Edema from fluid shifts may occur
- Skin may become warm and flushed (warm stage of septic shock)

Late Stage
- Cold, mottled, ashen, or cyanotic

Parameter
  Other

Early Stage
- Possible thirst
- Hypoactive bowel sounds that diminish
- Gastric motility
- Possible pupil dilation
- Pupils react equally to light

Middle Stage
- Possibly hypoactive or absent bowel sounds
- Paralytic ileus may occur
- GI ulcers may form
- Hematemesis or melena may occur
- Nausea, vomiting, or anorexia
- Possible body temperature decrease
- Muscle aches
- Lactic acid accumulation

Late Stage
- Multi-system organ failure
- Immune system collapse
- Coagulation cascade impairment
- Disseminated intravascular coagulation

CONTINUOUS MIXED VENOUS OXYGEN SATURATION (SvO_2) MONITORING

- Performed with a fiberoptic oximetry pulmonary artery catheter that is connected with a monitor that gives a continuous digital display of the percentage of mixed venous oxygen saturation.
- The fiberoptic carries red and infrared light from the monitor to the distal tip of the catheter. The light that emanates from this fiber scatters off of the red blood cells that are flowing past the tip, and the backscattered light is received by another fiber. The SvO_2 measurement is derived from the analyzing of the intensities of the light.
- SvO_2 monitoring often provides the first early warning signs that the patient's oxygenation status is deteriorating. Changes occur quickly and are present prior to arterial compromise. This can reduce the frequency for arterial blood gas sampling.
  - Normal SvO_2 is 70-80%
  - Normal PvO_2 is 40 mm Hg
  - AV difference = $SaO_2 - SvO_2$ [normal is 20]
  - AV oxygen content difference = $CaO_2 - CvO_2$ [normal is 5]

PULMONARY ARTERY CATHETERS

A pulmonary artery (PA) catheter is a special catheter with several lumens including a proximal (right atrium) port, a distal (PA) port, a balloon port, a port to connect with the thermistor, and sometimes 1 or more lumens for IV fluid administration.

A PA catheter is usually inserted through the subclavian vein but may be inserted femorally or brachially. Using sterile technique, place the catheter percutaneously and thread through the right atrium, the right ventricle and into the pulmonary artery, where the end floats with the vessel. A PA line is placed for obtaining reading of PA pressures, cardiac output measurement, mixed venous blood sampling. It is used with an oximetry catheter to obtain continuous readings of mixed venous oxygen saturation.

Several pressures can be noted with the PA catheter—PA systolic, diastolic, and mean pressures, pulmonary capillary wedge pressure (PCWP), right atrial pressure (CVP) as well as many measurements that are calculated using these values.

When a PA line is initially inserted, note the insertion length by the markings on the catheter. (Each wide mark is 50 cm; each single thin mark is 10 cm.) Obtain a tracing of the PA and PCWP waveforms for comparison later. Performance of the square waveform test will help differentiate the source of monitoring problems.

While quickly putting pigtail on a flush device and releasing, observe monitor for a squared waveform. If the waveform is squared, any monitoring problem will probably be due to the PA catheter or the patient. If the waveform is rounded or curved, the problem lies in the monitor or transducer.

To obtain the PCWP, or "wedge" pressure, insert 0.5 to 1.5 cc of air via the balloon port, which inflates the balloon at the end of the PA catheter. This enables the catheter to float out and wedge in a branch of the pulmonary vascular free, which gives an indirect measurement of the pressure in the pulmonary vein. This value can assist nurses and physicians to assess the patient's fluid and hemodynamic status. The balloon is NEVER left inflated for longer than 15 seconds at a time due to the possibility of pulmonary capillary rupture or infarction.

Cardiac output measurements can be performed with the thermodilution method. Using a closed system, inject 5-10 cc of iced or room temperature NS injectate rapidly (within 3-5 seconds) into the proximal port. The solution mixes with the blood travels through the vasculature to the thermistor where the temperature change is noted, along with conversion factors and time needed to travel the length of the catheter. This is computed as a measurement of L/min. Three measurements are performed and averaged, unless the patient has an irregular heart rhythm, and in that instance, 5 measurements may be performed. Each hospital will have its own procedure for this measurement

To ensure continuity in measurement, the transducer should be kept level at the patient's phlebostatic axis.

This axis is the crossing of two imaginary lines. One from a point with the 4th intercostal space joins the sternum to the side under the axilla. The other imaginary line runs halfway between the anterior and posterior surfaces of the chest. This axis should be marked on the patient so that each nurse will be leveling the bed and transducer to the same position each time. The phlebostatic axis correlates to the level of the right atrium and the O mark on the manometer or the transducer should be at this level.

At least 0.8 hrs, the PA line (as well as CVP arterial line, LA line, etc.) must be recalibrated. This involves opening the transducer to air and following the procedure designated by each hospital. This ensures accuracy with the line and the monitor.

TROUBLESHOOTING A PA MONITOR

PROBLEM
Dampening or disappearance of waveform

Interventions
- Turn stopcock off to the patient and flush the tubing.
- Check for kinks, especially at the insertion site.
- Check for air or blood in tubing.
- Make sure all stopcocks are open in the right direction and that connections are tight.
- Have the patient cough or turn in an effort to reposition the catheter to recover waveform.
- Check pressure on flush solution, and ascertain that flow rate is not impeded.
- Check for differentiation of problem location between catheter and system using fast flush (square waveform) check.
- Recalibrate.
- Check the transducer and change if necessary.
- Check the pressure monitor and change if necessary.
- Obtain chest x-ray for placement verification.

PROBLEM
Continuous RV waveform

Interventions
- Compare waveform with previous reading.
- Reposition the patient.
- Inflate balloon in an attempt to float the catheter into the PA.
- Obtain chest x-ray for placement verification.

PROBLEM
Continuous PCWP waveform

Interventions
- Reposition the patient.
- Have the patient cough or turn.
- Check inflation port and make sure the balloon is deflated.
- Aspirate blood from PA lumen to ascertain if blood is arterialized. If so, blood will be obtained with difficulty and most likely catheter is wedged.
- If all other measures fail, pull back the catheter cautiously 1-3 cm, just until PCWP waveform disappears if allowed per hospital policy.
- Notify MD.

PROBLEM
Fluctuation of waveform

Interventions
- Suspect catheter whip or respiratory deviations.
- This may require manipulation of the catheter to obtain optimal pattern.
- Check catheter markings for placement.

PROBLEM
Inability to obtain PCWP

Interventions
- Check the waveform to ascertain location of catheter.
- Verify that placement of catheter has not changed by observing markings on catheter.

- Reposition the patient.
- Check resistance to balloon inflation to rule out balloon rupture.
- Inflate the balloon to advance into the PA branch once rupture has been ruled out.
- Check syringe for leaks.
- Use PA diastolic pressure if relationship between PAD and PCWP have been consistent.
- Notify physician.

PROBLEM
Air or blood in setup
Interventions
- Tighten all connections.
- Check tubing and transducer for fractures.
- Aspirate from the stopcock if a clot is suspected.
- Flush system away from the patient to clear.
- Change transducer tubing.
- Check pressure on flush solution.
- Check fluid level of flush solution.

PROBLEM
Increased ventricular ectopy/irritability
Interventions
- Check for RV migration and fluctuation of waveform.
- Administer anti-arrhythmic medications prn.
- Obtain chest x-ray for catheter placement verification.

PROBLEM
Changes in data not correlating with patient's physical condition

Interventions
- Recalibrate, making sure level of transducer is positioned at patient's phlebostatic axis.
- Observe waveform.
- Flush line.

CARDIAC MONITORING AND PACEMAKERS

284 Cardiac Monitoring and Pacemakers

TABLE OF CONTENTS

Leads 286
Modified Chest Lead 287
Probability of SVT vs. VT 288
QRS Complexes 290
EKG Wave Patterns 291
Heart Rate Calculation 293
EKG Rhythm Determination 294
Dangerous Premature Ventricular Contractions 295
Normals on 12-Lead EKG 295
EKG Rhythm Determination 296
Heart Murmurs and Conditions that Cause Them 301
Einthoven's Triangle 303
Axis Determination 304
EKG Changes 305
EKG Changes in Myocardial Infarction 306
Causes of Hypertrophy 309
AV Conduction Defects 309
EKG Data and Changes with Certain Conditions 310
Events in the Cardiac Cycle 314
Basic Parts of a Pacemaker 315
Pacemaker Rates 317
Pacemaker Terminology 317
Pacemakers 324
Troubleshooting Pacemakers 326
Auscultation of Heart Sounds 328
Procedure for Immediate Return of
Post-op Cardiac Patient 330
Intra-Aortic Balloon Therapy 333
IABP Terminology 335
IABP Waveform 339
Symptoms of Cardiac Tamponade 340
Cardiac Catheterization Complications 341
Percutaneous Transluminal Coronary
Angioplasty Complications 341
Causes of Coronary Artery Reocclusion
after PTCA 342
Wolff-Parkinson-White Syndrome 342
Wellen's Syndrome 343

HEART
Chambers of the Heart

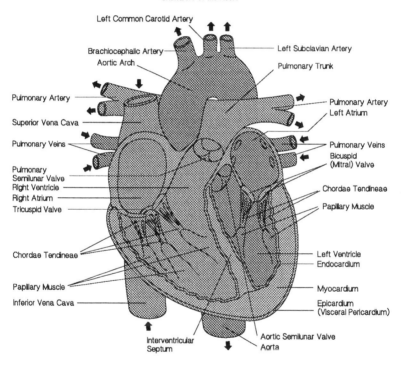

Anterior View

CARDIAC MONITORING LEADS

Lead	Negative	Positive	Ground
I	R arm	L arm	L leg
II	R arm	L leg	L arm
III	L arm	L leg	R arm
AVR		R arm	
AVL		L arm	
AVF		L leg	

PLACEMENT OF LEADS

V1 4th intercostal space, right sternal border
V2 4th intercostal space, left sternal border
V3 Halfway between V2 and V4
V4 5th intercostal space, left midclavicular line
V5 5th intercostal space, left anterior axillary line
V6 5th intercostal space, left midaxillary line

Lewis Lead	useful in seeing rhythms where atrial activity is questionable
R arm negative	2nd intercostal space, right sternal border
L arm positive	4th intercostal space, right eternal border
L leg ground	4th intercostal space, left eternal border

MODIFIED CHEST LEAD 1 (MCL$_1$)

(Useful in differentiating ventricular ectopy bundle branch blocks.)

Similar to V$_1$ lead

Positive electrode	4th intercostal space, right sternal border
Negative electrode	left clavicular mid sternal area
Ground electrode	below the mid right clavicular area
RBBB:	"right is upright"
	rSR' pattern [upward deflection]
LBBB	"left is lower"
	negative QS or rs pattern [downward deflection]
RV ectopy	QRS complex downward, usually RS pattern
LV ectopy	QRS complex upright, usually QR, qR or R; rabbit ear configuration has a taller left "ear" than the right Rsr'

PROBABILITY OF SVT vs. VT

QRS Configuration in Lead V_1		High Probability
Monophasic R	⋀	VT
Monophasic QS	⊤⋁⊤	55% SVT
Biphasic RS	—⋀⋁—	VT
Biphasic QR	⋁⋀—	VT
Biphasic rS	⋁	VT

Triphasic rSR' or rR'	∿ ∿	SVT
Taller left rabbit ear	∿	VT
Taller right rabbit ear	∿	61% VT

QRS Configuration in Lead V₆		**High Probability**
Monophasic QS	V	VT
Biphasic QR	∿	VT
Biphasic rS	∿	90% VT

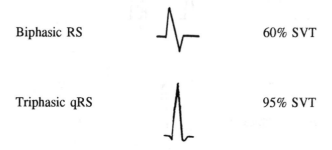

Biphasic RS — 60% SVT

Triphasic qRS — 95% SVT

QRS COMPLEXES

If there are several positive and/or negative deflections, the larger amplitudes are denoted by a capital letter and the smaller amplitudes are denoted with a small letter. In the case of having a second wave of the same type, it will be denoted with ′ (prime), such as, rsr′.

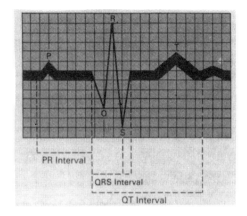

EKG WAVE PATTERNS

P wave—represents atrial depolarization

Q wave—first initial downward deflection before a positive deflection *(not always present)*

R wave—first positive upward deflection

S wave—first downward deflection following a positive wave

T wave—represents ventricular repolarization

PR interval—represents atrial depolarization and conduction time through the AV node

ST segment—represents the beginning of ventricular repolarization

PR segment—represents the delay at the AV node

QRS complex—represents ventricular depolarization

QT interval—represents the time required for depolarization and repolarization to take place: the time for repolarization is proportional to the heart rate and varies for men, women and children.

Cardiac Monitoring and Pacemakers

Isoelectric Line—a straight line representing the absence of electrical activity or equal amounts of movement away from the particular electrode during depolarization.

NORMAL MEASUREMENTS

P wave: < 3 mm high
Q wave: < 0.04 sec wide or < ⅓ of R wave height
R wave: < 13 mm high
PR interval: 0.12 to 0.20 seconds
QRS duration: < 0.10 seconds
QT interval: usually < 0.44 sec

Formula to correct QT for heart rate:

Corrected QT QT_c = $\dfrac{\text{measured QT (sec)}}{\sqrt{R-R \text{ interval (sec)}}}$

INHERENT RATE RANGES

SA node 60 to 100
AV junction 40 to 60
Ventricle 20 to 40

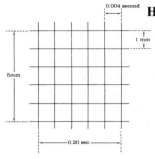

How The Time Is Measured

Each small box = 0.04 sec
Each large box = 0.20
Five large boxes = 1 sec
Five large boxes = 1" graph paper
Each small box = 1 mm sq
5 mm = 0.5 mV

HEART RATE CALCULATION

The heart rate can be approximately determined in several ways by using an EKG rhythm strip

Method A: Count the number of R waves in a 6-second rhythm strip and multiply by 10.

(If the heart rhythm is regular, the following methods will be accurate.)

Method B: Count the number of small squares between two consecutive R waves and divide into 1500

Method C: Count the number of large squares between two consecutive waves and divide into 300

Method D: Use the scale below; this scale represents the distance in large squares between two consecutive R waves:

- 1 large square = 300 beats per minute
- 2 large squares = 150 beats per minute
- 3 large squares = 100 beats per minute
- 4 large squares = 75 beats per minute
- 5 large squares = 60 beats per minute
- 6 large squares = 50 beats per minute
- 7 large squares = 43 beats per minute
- 8 large squares = 38 beats per minute
- 9 large squares = 33 beats per minute

EKG RHYTHM DETERMINATION

Determination of rhythm can be accomplished by utilizing the following steps:

Rate

Normal	=	60 to 100 (sinus)
Bradycardia	=	< 60 (junctional or nodal 40-60 rate, ventricular 20-40 rate)
Tachycardia	=	> 100

Rhythm

Normal	=	regular R-R intervals
Abnormal	=	irregularly irregular or regularly irregular R-R intervals

P-R Interval

Normal	=	0.10 to 0.20 seconds (sinus)
1st degree AV block	=	greater than 0.20 seconds
Atrial	=	less than 0.10 seconds

QRS Duration

Normal	=	< 0.10 seconds

Bundle Branch Block = > 0.10 seconds

P waves

Normal	=	P waves present, normal, and occur before each QRS complex
Inverted	=	impulse originates in atria or nodal area

Variable Configuration = wandering pacemaker

Absent	=	Sinoatrial arrest, SA block, atrial fibrillation

DANGEROUS PREMATURE VENTRICULAR CONTRACTIONS

- Multifocal PVCs
- VT
- Greater than 6 PVCs per minute
- Torsades de pointes
- Couplets or salvoes
- R-on-T phenomenon
- Bigeminy, Trigeminy, Quadrigeminy

NORMALS ON 12-LEAD EKG

Limb Leads
- Lead I: QRS and T upright
- Lead II: QRS and T upright
- Lead III: QRS and T upright

Augmented Unipolar Leads
- Lead AVR: QRS and T downward
- Lead AVL: QRS and T upright
- Lead AVF: QRS and T upright

Precordial (chest) leads

Moving from V, toward V_6, normal R wave progression means that R waves become progressively larger and S waves become progressively smaller, R should be equiphasic by V_3.

EKG RHYTHM DETERMINATION

Item	NSR	Sinus Bradycardia	Sinus Tachycardia	Sinus Arrythmia
P wave	Normal	Normal	Normal	Normal
QRS	Normal	Normal	Normal	Normal
P: QRS	1:1	1:1	1:1	1:1
Rate A Rate V	60-100 60-100	40-60 40-60	100-180 100-180	60-100 60-100
Rhythm	Regular	Regular	Regular	Irregular
Other information				Varying R-R interval related to respiration pattern

EKG RHYTHM DETERMINATION

Item	Premature Atrial Contractions	Multifocal Atrial Tachycardia	Atrial Tachycardia	Atrial Fibrillation	Atrial Flutter
P wave	Different from normal	Variable	Difficult to find	"f" waves	Flutter waves
QRS	Normal	Normal	Normal	Normal	Normal
P: QRS	1:1	1:1	1:1	1:1	1:1
Rate A Rate V	Variable usually normal	100-250 100-250	150-250 150-250	A-up to 700 V-variable	A-200-350 V-variable
Rhythm	Mildly irregular	Irregular	Regular	Irregular	Regular or irregular
Other information	Intermittently irregular due to ectopy, compensatory pause occurs after beat but is not a full pause	Associated with COPD	R-R interval regular or variable if AV block occurs PR shortened		Sawtooth pattern, will probably change to atrial fibrillation

EKG RHYTM DETERMINATION

Item	Sinus Block	Sinus Arrest	Wandering Atrial Pacemaker	Junctional
P wave	None	None	Variable configurations	Inverted, before, in or after QRS
QRS	None	None	Normal	Normal
P: QRS			1:1	1:1
Rate	Variable, usually 40-70	Variable, usually 40-70	60-100 may be slow	40-60
Rhythm	Irregular due to missed beat, otherwise regular	Irregular due to missed beat, otherwise regular	Regular	Regular
Other information	Interval before and after pause is 2 × normal intervals; no PR during block	Long pause after preceding conducted beat; R-R varies; no PR during arrest	R-R irregular due to pacemaker site shifting; PR may vary slightly	R-R regular

EKG RHYTHM DETERMINATION

Item	Premature Junctional Contraction	Accelerated Junctional	Junctional Tachycardia	Paroxysmal Supraventricular Tachycardia	Premature Ventricular Contraction
P wave	Inverted before, in, or after QRS	Inverted before, in, or after QRS	Inverted before, in, or after QRS	May be similar to sinus P	None visible
QRS	Normal	Normal	Normal	Normal	Wide, bizarre
P: QRS	Variable	1:1	1:1	1:1	
Rate A Rate V	60-100	60-100	100-160	100-180	Variable
Rhythm	Irregular due to ectopy	Regular	Regular	Irregular	Irregular due to ectopy
Other information	May have short compensatory pause after ectopic beat	R-R regular		Sudden onset and cessation of SVT	Compensatory pause with R-R= 2 sinus intervals

EKG RHYTHM DETERMINATION

Item	1° AV Block	2° AV block Type I	2° AV block, Type II	3° AV block (CHB)	VT	VF
P wave	Normal	Normal	Normal	PR variable none	None visible	None
QRS	Normal	Normal	Usually widened	Wide, may be normal	Wide, bizarre	None
P: QRS	1:1	p> QRS variable	p. QRS variable	p > QRS no relation	No ratio	None
Rate V	60-100	40-60	40-60	30-50	140-250	None
Rhythm	Regular	Irregular	Irregular or regular	A & V rhythms regular but independent of each other	Regular or irregular	
Other Information	Prolonged PR	Progressive prolongation of PR until a beat is dropped	Sudden blocking of sinus impulses without prolongation of PR		R-R mostly regular with no association with P	

HEART MURMURS AND CONDITIONS THAT CAUSE THEM

Condition	Timing	Place and Duration	Pitch	Location	Intensity	Quality	Radiation
Mitral insufficiency	Systolic	Pansystolic/ ejection; if mild, late systolic	High	Apex	I-V/VI	Plateau	Left axilla
Tricuspid insufficiency	Systolic	Pansystolic/ ejection	Medium	LLSB	I-V/VI	Plateau	Right eternal border
Aortic stenosis	Systolic	Midsystolic	Medium	2 RICS	Varies	Crescendo-decrescendo	Neck, upper back, right carotid, apex
IHSS	Systolic	Ejection	High	2-4 RICS	Varies	Crescendo	Neck, upper back, apex
Pulmonic stenosis	Systolic	Midsystolic	Medium	2 LICS	III-IV/VI	Crescendo	Left side of neck
Ventricular septal defect	Systolic	Pansystolic/ ejection	High	LLSB	Varies	Plateau	Widely

HEART MURMURS AND CONDITIONS THAT CAUSE THEM

Condition	Timing	Place and Duration	Pitch	Location	Intensity	Quality	Radiation
Coarctation of aorta	Systolic	Ejection	Medium	Left midback between scapulas	Varies	Crescendo	Neck
Mitral stenosis	Diastolic	Midsystolic/ presystolic	Low	Apex	I-II/VI	Crescendo	None
Tricuspid stenosis	Diastolic	Early diastolic	High	4 LICS	Varies	Decrescendo	Apex, xiphoid
Aortic insufficiency	Diastolic	Early diastolic	High	3-4 LICS 2 RICS	I-VI/VI	Decrescendo	Apex, left sternal border
Pulmonic insufficiency	Diastolic	Early Diastolic	High	2 LICS	Varies	Decrescendo	Apex
Patent ductus arteriosus, aortic atrial shunt	Systolic-diastolic	Continuous	High	2 LICS	Varies	Varies	Neck

EINTHOVEN'S TRIANGLE

Einthoven's triangle is a hypothetical triangle formed by the arms and legs with the heart at the center. The normal flow of current is from a negative (−) to a positive (+). If an impulse travels from − to +, it is a positive deflection. If the impulse goes from + to −, it is a negative deflection.

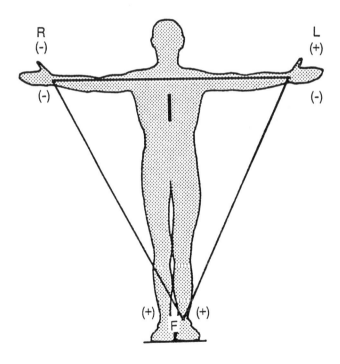

AXIS DETERMINATION
Normal Axis is -30 to + 110 degrees

To determine the axis, find the most biphasic lead in the 12 lead EKG. Using the graph, find the perpendicular lead to the biphasic lead. Depending on the deflection of the complex, go to the negative (downward deflection) or positive (upward deflection) end of the graph line for the angle.

Left Axis Deviation

Lead I upward deflection

Lead AVR downward deflection

Extreme Right Axis Deviation

Lead 1 downward deflection

Lead AVF downward deflection

Right Axis Deviation

Lead I downward deflection

Lead AVL upward deflection

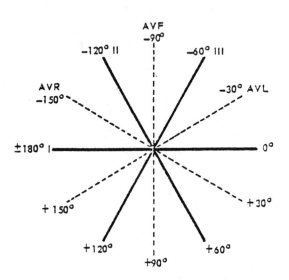

Left Axis Deviation	Right Axis Deviation
Left ventricular hypertrophy	Right ventricular hypertrophy
Left anterior hemiblock	Dextrocardia
Left bundle branch block	Right bundle branch block
Inferior MI	
WPW syndrome	Left posterior hemiblock
Pregnancy	Left ventricular ectopy
Ascites	COPD
Tumors	Pulmonary emboli/infarcts
Elderly or obese patients	Young, tall, or thin patients (infants are born with RAD; then it changes)

EKG CHANGES
- T wave inversion—ischemia
- ST elevation—injury
- Q waves—necrosis, death

EKG CHANGES IN MYOCARDIAL INFARCTION

Wall Affected	Leads	Possible EKG Changes	Artery Involved
Inferior	II, III, AVF	Q, ST, T	Right Coronary (RCA)
Lateral	I, AVL, V_5, V_6	Q, ST, T	Circumflex (Cx)
Anterior	V_1, V_2, I, AVL	Q, ST, T loss of R wave progression	Left anterior descending (LAD)
Posterior	V_1, V_2, (opposite)	R greater than S, ST depression, elevated T wave (reciprocal changes)	RCA, Circumflex (Cx)
Apical	V_3-V_6	Q, ST, T loss of R wave progression	LAD, RCA
Septal	V_1-V_2	Q, ST, T	Septal
Anterolateral	I, AVL, V_1-V_6	Q, ST, T	LAD, Circumflex (Cx)
Anteroseptal	V_1-V_4	Q, ST, T loss of septal R wave in V_1	LAD

EKG CHANGES IN MYOCARDIAL INFARCTION

Wall Affected	Leads	Possible EKG Changes	Artery Involved
Non Q-wave	Any of the above	ST, T for more than 3 days with enzyme changes	
Right Ventricular	V_1, RV_3, RV_4	Q, ST, T	RCA

Intrinsicoid deflection = ventricular activation time= (VAT) onset of QRS to the peak of the R wave; reflects time required for peak voltage

Right atrial abnormality (or hypertrophy)
- Tall, peaked P waves in Leads II, III, AVF (> 2.5 mm)
- Large biphasic or inverted P wave in V_1
- P pulmonale

Left atrial abnormality (or hypertrophy)
- Wide, notched P in lead II (> 0.12 sec)
- Biphasic P wave in V_1 with a broad negative phase, > 0.04 sec
- P mitrale

Right ventricular hypertrophy (RVH)
- Right axis deviation of + 110° or more
- Deep S wave in V_5-V_6, I, and AVL
- P in V_1 + S in V_6 11 mm or more
- rSR' in V_1 with R' ≥ to 11 mm

- qR in V_1
- R wave > S in V_1
- S wave > R in V_6
- P pulmonale (P greater than 2.5 mm in height in II, III, AVF)
- Intrinsicoid deflection in $V_1 \geq 0.035$

Left Ventricular Hypertrophy (LVH)

- R wave in lead V_5 or $V_6 \pm$ S wave in lead V_1 > 35 mm
- R wave in lead I + S wave in lead III > 25 mm
- R wave in lead I > an 15 mm
- R wave in lead AVL > 11 mm
- R wave in lead AVF > 20 mm
- Intrinsicoid deflection in V_3-V_6 > 0.05
- Left axis deviation (in 50% of patients)
- QRS and T are different angles on axis determination
- S wave in lead V_1 or V_2 30 mm or more
- Non-specific ST and T wave changes

CAUSES OF HYPERTROPHY

Right Ventricular Hypertrophy	Left Ventricular Hypertrophy
Hypoxia	Hypertension
COPD	Aortic regurgitation/stenosis
Pulmonary hypotension	Mitral regurgitation
Chronic left ventricular failure	Leaky valve
Tricuspid regurgitation	Atrial dsyrhythmias
Pulmonary regurgitation/Stenosis	Athletes
Atrial—or ventricular—septal defect	

AV CONDUCTION DEFECTS

First degree AV block:
  PR > 0.20 sec, due to delay of impulse at AV junction

Second degree AV block, type I:
  (Mobitz I, Wenchebach)—PR is progressively lengthened until a sinus beat fails to conduct through the AV node, and a QRS complex is dropped. R-R interval decreases as PR increases; P-P interval remains unchanged

Second degree AV block, type II
  (Mobitz II)—at intervals, one or more p waves do not conduct through the AV node to the ventricles, R-R varies: P-P unchanged, PR unchanged.

Third degree AV block
  (Complete heart block)—there is no conduction of impulses through the AV node: may have sinus impulses and junctional or ventricular escape rhythms

that are completely independent of each other. R-R is regular, P-P is regular, PR not regular

EKG DATA AND CHANGES WITH CERTAIN MEDICAL CONDITIONS

Right Bundle Branch Block (RBBB)
- rSR' in V_1 (or V_2 or AVR)
- qRS in V_6
- Wide QRS > 0.12 sec
- Wide terminal S wave in leads I, AVL, V_5, and V_6
- Secondary ST and T wave changes

Left Bundle Branch Block (LBBB)
- Wide QRS > 0.12 sec
- Negative deflection, often notched, in V_1
- Positive deflection with broad notched R wave in V_6
- No Q wave in leads I, AVL, V_6
- Notched QRS in leads, I, AVL, V_6
- ST and T wave changes
- Prolonged activation time of the septum and the left ventricle

Left Anterior Hemiblock (LAHB)
- More common than LPHB
- Left axis deviation of $-45°$ or more
- qR in lead I, AVL
- rS in lead II, III, AVF
- QRS at upper limits of normal

Left Posterior Hemiblock (LPHB)
- Rare, with high mortality; usually seen with severe cardiac disease
- Right axis deviation of + 120° or more
- qR in lead II, III, AVF
- rS in lead I, AVL
- RV hypertrophy should be ruled out

Pulmonary Hypertension
- Peaked P waves in leads II, III, AVF
- Large R wave in V_1-V_3
- ST changes
- Inverted T wave
- Low voltage
- Right axis deviation
- Right ventricular hypertrophy

Cor Pulmonale
- Tall, peaked P waves in leads II, III, AVF
- T wave inversion
- ST changes
- Right axis deviation
- Right ventricular hypertrophy
- Low voltage
- Intraventricular conduction defect

Pulmonary Embolism
- ST and T wave changes
- Sinus tachycardia
- Peaked P waves
- Atrial fibrillation

- Large S waves in lead I
- Q wave in lead III
- Inverted T wave in lead III
- Right bundle branch block

Acute Pericarditis
- ST segment elevation in 2-3 limb leads
- ST segment elevation in precordial leads
- PR segment depression in V_1, AVR
- Widespread T wave inversion

Digitalis Toxicity
- ST sagging
- Flattened T waves
- Shortened QT
- SVT, PSVT, PVCs, VT, A, F, B
- SA and AV blocks

Hyperkalemia
- High, peaked T waves
- Prolonged PR with flattened P waves as potassium increases
- ST elevation
- Widened QRS
- Possible heart blocks

Hypokalemia
- Flattened, inverted T waves
- U waves prominent
- ST segment depression

- PR may be prolonged
- Prolonged QT

Hypercalcemia
- Shortened QT
- Widened QRS
- Inverted T waves
- Shortened or absent ST segment

Hypocalcemia or hypermagnesemia
- Prolonged QT
- Prolonged isoelectric ST segment

Tall T waves are seen with these conditions:
- Infarction
- Potassium excess
- Ischemia
- Ventricular overload
- Use of antipsychotic drugs
- CVA

EVENTS IN THE CARDIAC CYCLE

Cycle initiated by depolarization of SA node (*P wave on EKG*)

Contraction of the atria

- Causing a rise in pressure and responsible for the A wave on CVP
- 4th heart sound
- Ventricles are in diastole
- Depolarizing stimulus arrives at the AV node and spreads quickly through the bundle of His and the Purkinje fibers (*QRS on EKG*)

Contraction of the ventricles:

- The first phase of ventricular systole is called the isovolumetric contraction (represents the pressure increases without blood moving into or out of ventricles.)
- First heart sound (S_1) begins as the pressure increases and the AV valves close. This occurs when the **c wave** on CVP is produced. As the pressure increases, the aortic valve opens, and blood is ejected into the aorta rapidly. As the blood is pumped out, the pressure decreases and the aortic valve closes, causing the 2nd heart sound (S_2).
- Apex beat
- Repolarization begins (*T wave on EKG*)

Relaxation of the ventricles: systole ends

- When aortic valve closes, the left ventricular pressure increases and the isovolumetric relaxation phase begins and is responsible for the **v wave** on CVP.
- Third heart sound
- Cycle restarts

PACEMAKERS

BASIC PARTS OF A PACEMAKER

Output or MA dial: controls the amount of current delivered to the endocardium or epicardium; the amount of energy required to elicit myocardial depolarization: (Usually 3-5 MA)

Rate dial: determines the rate in bpm (beats per minute) at which the stimulus or current is to be delivered. (Usually 50-80)

Sensitivity dial: produces the degree that the pacing system "sees" or senses the signals. The voltage required to deliver the current (MA); in maximum clockwise position, this provides demand or synchronous pacing, in maximum counter clockwise position, this provides fixed rate or asynchronous. Newer pacemakers use digital controls rather than dials.

On-Off switch: turns the pacemaker on and off; the circular area to the right of this switch has a small black raised knob that must be pushed in order to turn the pacemaker off. This is a safety feature so that the pacemaker cannot be accidently turned off. *(See the pacemaker illustration on the following page.)*

316 *Cardiac Monitoring and Pacemakers*

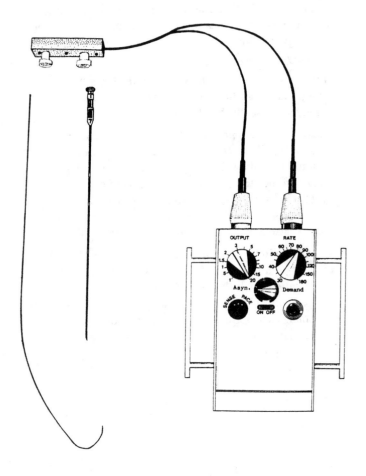

PACEMAKER RATES

Fixed rate pacing: (ASYNCHRONOUS): The heart is stimulated at a fixed rate that is preset, independent of the heart's own electrical activity. Should the heart's own rhythm compete with that of the pacer, it may precipitate ventricular fibrillation.

Non-competitive pacing: (SYNCHRONOUS) *Demand* or *ventricular-inhibited,* the pacemaker is inhibited as long as the inherent rate is faster than the preset pacer rate. *Standby* or *ventricular-activated*—the firing of the pacemaker is triggered by each QRS and delivered immediately, if the spontaneous QRS fails, the pacemaker will discharge.

PACEMAKER TERMINOLOGY

Ablation—the removal, isolation or destruction of cardiac tissue or pathways involved with arrhythmias; may be achieved by a variety of surgical and electrode catheter techniques.

Action potential—the changes in electrical potential generated by the cell membrane following stimulation of muscle or nerve cells. The action potential has five phases, phase 0 is the period of rapid depolarization and the reversal of polarity from negative to slightly positive. The remaining four phases are concerned with returning the cell to its resting membrane potential where it remains until the next stimulus.

Activity threshold—the level of activity which must be exceeded before activity detecting, rate responsive pacemakers will increase pacing rates.

Ampere (amp)—the amount of electrical current flowing past a point in a conductor when one volt of potential is applied across one ohm of resistance. In pacing, these currents are so small that they are expressed in milliamperes, or one-thousandth of an amp (ma).

Atrial Tracking—a pacing mode in which the ventricles are paced in synchrony with sensed atrial events.

A-V Interval—the period of time between an atrial event (sensed or paced) and a paced ventricular event when using a dual-chamber pacemaker

Bipolar—having two poles, or electrodes, both of which are located externally to the pulse generator, usually in the heart. (A bipolar pacing lead has two electrodes: a small tip electrode through which the heart is usually stimulated, and a ring electrode, located several millimeters proximal to the tip electrode which completes the electrical circuit. During pacing, the current flow is between these two electrodes and they also serve to sense spontaneous heart activity.)

Blanking period—the interval of time during which the pacemaker cannot sense any events.

Burst pacing—the delivery of rapid, multiple electrical stimuli. This type of pacing is typically used to interrupt a fast heart rate.

Capture—depolarization of the atria and/or ventricles by an electrical stimulus delivered by an artificial pacemaker. One-to-one capture occurs when each electrical stimulus causes a corresponding depolarization.

Cross talk—the phenomenon that can occur in dual chamber pacemakers in which a stimulus from the atrial lead is sensed by the ventricular lead, or vice versa, resulting in an inappropriate pacemaker response such as inhibition or resetting of the refractory period

Dual chamber pacing—pacing in both the atria and the ventricles to artificially restore the natural contraction sequence of the heart

Electrogram (EGM)—in pacing, the recording of the cardiac waveforms as taken at the lead site within the heart.

Electromagnetic interference—radiated or conducted energy—either electrical or magnetic—which can interfere with or disrupt the function of a pulse generator in the demand mode.

Electrophysiologic study—invasive study of the electrical behavior of the heart done to diagnose and study arrhythmias of the heart.

End-of-life (EOL)—the point at which a pacemaker signals that it should be replaced because its battery is nearing depletion.

Escape Interval—the time between a paced or sensed cardiac event and the subsequent pacing stimulus of a pulse generator.

Exit block—failure of a pacemaker to capture the heart because the stimulation threshold exceeds the output of the pacemaker

Fusion beat—a spontaneous cardiac depolarization which occurs coincidentally with a paced depolarization and produce a collision waveform

Hysteresis—a pacing parameter which usually allows a longer escape interval after a sensed event, giving the heart a greater opportunity to beat on its own. If the hysteresis period elapses and no natural depolarization occurs, the pulse generator will revert to its faster rate and begin pacing at this rate.

Impedance—the total opposition that a circuit presents to an alternating electrical current.

Implantable pulse generator—a pacemaker that is used for permanent pacing and is placed inside a pocket under the skin with the leads positioned in or on the heart.

Impulse—the term used to describe the electrical stimulus delivered by a pacemaker.

Lead—in a pacemaker system, the lead is composed of the wire or wires that carry electrical signals to and from the heart, a connector pin, and stimulating/sensing electrodes.

Lead active fixation—a packing lead which has some mechanism at the lead tip which can be embedded in heart tissue, making displacement less likely to occur.

Lead, atrial—a lead that is designed for use in or on the atria; because of the nature of atrial tissue, endocardial atrial leads often are shaped as a "j" to ensure fixation in the atria

Lead, endocardial—(sometimes called a transvenous lead) a pacing lead which is passed transvenously and lodged in either the right atrium or right ventricle

Lead, low threshold — a term that describes leads that provide relatively low pacing thresholds

Lead, myocardial—a lead with an electrode designed to be attached to the outside of the heart

Lead, permanent—any lead intended for implantation and long-term use

Lead, steroid eluting—term used to describe an implanted lead that elutes an anti-inflammatory drug through the electrode and maintains low pacing thresholds.

The ICU Quick Reference 321

Lead, temporary—a lead intended for short-term use which is placed either epicardially or transvenously and is usually used with an external pacemaker

Lead, transvenous—a lead that is passed through a vein.

Lead, ventricular—a lead that is designed for use in or on the ventricle

Membrane potential—the voltage difference existing between the inside and the outside of the cell membrane of those cells which have not been depolarized

NBG code—five letter codes for identifying pulse generators and pacing modes developed by the North American Society of Pacing and Electrophysiology and the British Pacing and Electrophysiology Group. The first letter represent the heart chamber paced, the second letter represents the heart chamber sensed, the third letter represents the mode of response from the pulse generator, the fourth letter represents the pulse generator's programmability and/or rate responsiveness, and the fifth letter represents any special anti-tachycardia function of the pulse generator.

Overdrive pacing—pacing the heart at a rate faster than the patient's own intrinsic rhythm, usually used to suppress a tachydysrhythmia, to gain electrical control of the heart, or to suppress PVCs

Oversensing—inhibition of a pacemaker by events other than those which the pacemaker was designed to sense, such as myopotentials, electromagnetic interference, T- wave, crosstalk, etc.

Pacemaker, artificial—a device which provides timed electrical stimuli to the heart, consisting of the pulse generator and the lead that carries the electrical impulses between the pulse generator and the heart.

Pacemaker, asynchronous—a pacemaker that stimulates at a fixed preset rate, independently of the electrical and/or mechanical activity of the heart

Pacemaker, demand (or inhibited)— a pacemaker that, after sensing a spontaneous depolarization, withholds its pacing stimulus

Pacemaker, atrial synchronous—a dual chamber pacemaker which senses atrial activity and paces only in the ventricle

Pacemaker, atrial synchronous, ventricular inhibited—a dual chamber pacemaker that senses in the atrium, and senses and paces in the ventricle

Pacemaker, A-V sequential—a dual chamber pacemaker that paces at a programmed rate in the atrium and senses and paces in the ventricle

Pacemaker, A-V Universal—a dual chamber pacemaker which can pace and sense in both the atria and the ventricles

Pacemaker, rate responsive—a pacemaker that can change the pacing rate in response to detected changes in the body to meet the metabolic need for greater blood flow.

Pacemaker, external—any pulse generator intended to be worn outside the body and used for temporary pacing

Pulse width—the duration of the pacing pulse expressed in milliseconds

Reversion—automatic suspension of the pacemaker's inhibition function in the presence of certain types of electrical activity; the pacemaker will continue to pace, rather than inhibit in the presence of continuous electromagnetic interference

Sensing threshold—the minimum atrial or ventricular intracardiac signal amplitude required to inhibit or trigger a demand pacemaker

Underdrive pacing—pacing at a rate below the tachycardia rate, for the purpose of interrupting the heart's tachy circuit with randomly timed stimuli so as to gain control of the heart and restore its natural rhythm

Undersensing—failure of the pacemaker to sense the P wave or R wave that may cause the pacemaker to emit inappropriately timed impulses

From Medtronic Pacing Glossary, Medtronic Informational Data. Used by permission of Medtronic, Inc,

PACEMAKERS

Increased sensitivity to pacing stimuli	Decreased sensitivity to pacing stimuli
• Hypokalemia	• Hyperkalemia
• Hypernatremia	• Hyponatremia
• Hypercalcemia	• Hypocalcemia
• Acidosis	• Alkalosis
• Digitalis toxicity	• Propranolol
• Steroids	• Verapamil
• Aldosterone antagonists	• Procainamide
• Exercise	• Quinidine
• Orthostasis	
• Hypoxia	
• Sympathetic stimulants	

Indications for Temporary Pacing

- Complete heart block with intermittent asystole
- Complete heart block with episodes of ventricular tachycardia or fibrillation
- Acute myocardial infarction complicated by complete heart block
- Symptomatic shifting heart block between second and third degree
- Bifascicular blocks
- Symptomatic bradydysrhythmias
- Cardiac arrest with ventricular asystole
- Sick sinus syndrome
- Digitalis toxicity
- Occurrence of heart block following cardiac surgery
- Permanent pacemaker replacement

- Prior to permanent pacemaker insertion

Measuring Stimulation Thresholds

- With the pacemaker turned off, set the output control at 5 MA.
- Set the rate control at least 10 beats above the patient's own intrinsic rate.
- Set the sensitivity control halfway between 1.5 mV and 3 mV.
- Connect the pacemaker to the patient and turn the pacemaker ON.
- Verify on the EKG the presence of 1:1 capture of the heart by a pacing stimulus.
- Gradually decrease the output current until 1:1. capture is lost.
- Gradually increase the output current to find the amplitude at which capture is regained.
- Reset the output control at 5 MA or a setting that is at least double the stimulation threshold found in previous step.

Measuring Sensitivity Thresholds

- Set the sensitivity control halfway between 1.5 mV and 3 mV.
- Set the rate control at least 10 beats below the patient's own intrinsic heart rate.
- Set the output control at 5 MA.
- The pacemaker should stop pacing and the sense indicator should start flashing as the unit senses naturally occurring R waves.
- Gradually turn the sensitivity control counter-clockwise until the pacemaker begins firing pacing stimuli and the pace indicator begins flashing, signifying the sensitivity threshold.

- Reset the sensitivity control 2 to 3 times more sensitive than the threshold level.

From Medtronic Informational Data. Used by permission of Medtronic, Inc.

TROUBLESHOOTING PACEMAKERS

SITUATION	POSSIBLE CAUSE	CORRECT APPROACH
Loss of pacer artifact	Pacemaker too sensitive	Reduce sensitivity (turn sensitivity dial to asynchronous or to a higher mV value
	Battery depletion	Change battery
	Loose, broken, disconnected wires	Change external pacemaker
	Short circuit of wire	Repair or replace pacing cath or the ground wire
Failure to capture without loss of pacing artifact	Catheter malposition	Increase output, reposition patient, reposition catheter
	Battery depletion	Change battery
	Electronic insulation break	Change external pacemaker repair insulation, change catheter
	Output setting too low	Increase output
Rate malfunction	Faulty external pacer	Change external pacemaker

TROUBLESHOOTING PACEMAKERS		
SITUATION	POSSIBLE CAUSE	CORRECT APPROACH
Loss of proper sensing	Catheter malposition; pacemaker not sensitive enough	Reposition catheter; increase sensitivity (turn dial to lower mv value)
	Faulty external pacer	Change external pacemaker
	Electrical interference caused reversion to a synchronous	Eliminate interference
Oversensing	Pacemaker too sensitive	Decrease sensitivity (turn sensitivity dial to asynchronous or higher mv value)
	Electrical interference	Eliminate interference, change external pacemaker
Pacemaker-induced arrhythmias	Output setting too high	Decrease output
	Electrical interference	Eliminate interference
	Altered threshold	Change mode or setting appropriate drugs
	Output too high	Reduce output
Stimulation of chest wall or diaphragm	Perforation; output too high	Change patient's position, reposition catheter; reduce output

From Medtronic Informational Data. Used by permission of Medtronic, Inc.

AUSCULTATION OF HEART SOUNDS

The bell of the stethoscope is best used for hearing low pitched sounds (S3, S4 ventricular murmurs). The diaphragm of the stethoscope is best used for hearing high-pitched sounds (S1, S2, clicks, snaps, stenotic valve murmurs)

S1
- First heart sound
- Associated with the turbulent blood flow against the closed mitral and tricuspid valves
- Followed by a quieter period called systole
- Softer sound than S2
- Heard loudest at the apex
- "Lub"

S2
- Second primary heart sound
- Associated with the turbulent blood flow against the closed aortic and pulmonic valves
- Followed by a quiet period called diastole
- Heard low at the base
- "Dub"

S3
- Ventricular gallop
- Can occur with 0.12-0.14 seconds after S2
- Associated with an increased volume load and increased pressure needed for complete ventricular filling
- Common in young people less than 20 years old and in athletes—abnormal in anyone else
- May signal CHF, left-to-right shunts, mitral or tricuspid insufficiency, cardiomyopathy
- Heard best over pulmonary valve with the bell of the stethoscope with patient in left lateral decubitus position. If the origin is in the left ventricle, it will be

heard best at the apex. If the origin is in the right ventricle, it will be heard best at the 3rd or 4th intercostal space at the left sternal border.
- "Ken-tuc-ky"

S4
- Atrial gallop
- Occurs either just before or during S1
- Associated with an increase in diastolic pressure or when ventricle is overloaded
- Related to atrial contractions
- Often occurs with hypertension, myocardial infarction, pulmonary hypertension, aortic or pulmonary stenosis, heart failure hyperthyroid crisis, or elderly due to decreased distensibility of left ventricle
- Always abnormal
- Best heard over pulmonary valve with the bell of the stethoscope
- "Ten-nes-see"

Ejection clicks
- Occur shortly after S1
- Can be heard at the apex and the base
- Aortic clicks can be heard at both the apex and the base, and occur with aortic dilation, hypertension, or with aortic valvular disease
- Pulmonary clicks can be heard over the pulmonic area, and occur with pulmonary artery dilation, pulmonary hypertension, or with pulmonary stenosis.

Murmurs
- Result from turbulent blood flow
- Graded on a scale of I to VI according to severity, with I being barely perceptible to VI being able to be heard without a stethoscope. The grade is written as a ratio showing the severity over the scale used.
- Systolic murmurs are those that occur with a pulse beat and are associated with conditions such as with mitral or tricuspid insufficiency, aortic or pulmonary stenosis, or septal rupture.

- Diastolic murmurs are those that do not occur with a pulse beat and are associated with conditions such as aortic or pulmonary regurgitation, or mitral or tricuspid stenosis.

PROCEDURE FOR IMMEDIATE RETURN OF POST-OP CARDIAC PATIENT

Obtain report on patient from surgical member:
- Pre-operative history
- Problems during surgery
- Procedure done
- Aortic cross clamp time
- Amount of blood and fluids given
- I&O
- Anesthetic agent used
- Estimated blood loss

Attach EKG monitor:
- Observe rate, rhythm, presence of dysrhythmias
- Treat problems as needed
- Obtain initial rhythm strip for baseline

Connect endotracheal tube to volume ventilator:
- Check for correct settings
- Check for ET placement and secure
- Auscultate breath sounds and heart sounds
- Suction as needed
- Observe for bilateral chest expansion, color, oxygenation
- Obtain oximetry reading

Check arterial line, pulmonary artery line, left atrial line:
- Calibrate and zero lines
- Check manual blood pressure for comparison
- Obtain vital signs, including temperature, pulse, respiration, BP, pulmonary artery pressures, PCWP, CO/CI, LA pressure, CVP, PVR, SVR, LVSWI, RVSWI, SV, SVI
- Obtain initial wave tracings for baseline

Establish IVs on infusion pumps
- Check all lines for patency
- Have multiple sites for emergency medicines
- Have line available for IV push drugs
- Evaluate all drips, making sure concentrations and flow rates are accurate
- Check orders for titration

Check pacemaker wires and connections
- Check all pacer settings; mode, rate, MA, sensitivity
- Ensure that pacer wires are connected and/or grounded
- Check that all lines, wires, etc. are secure with connections visible

Check urinary output
- Test urine for glucose and acetone as ordered
- Test urine for specific gravity as ordered
- Strict I&O q1h
- Check catheter for patency

332 Cardiac Monitoring and Pacemakers

Check mediastinal and pleural chest tubes
- Check connections to ensure no leakage
- Connect tubes with suction or gravity drainage as per orders
- Note drainage level and mark on tape affixed to bottle
- Check output q15-30 minutes × 2 hours, then q1-2 hours

Connect nasogastric tube to suction
- Check and confirm proper placement
- Irrigate prn
- Note amount, type and color of drainage
- Hematest any suspicious drainage for presence of blood
- Auscultate for bowel sounds
- Observe for abdominal distention

Perform a head-to-toe assessment
- Withhold sedating agents until level of responsiveness is established, then administer sedation and/or analgesics

Assist with procedures ordered
- EKG
- CXR
- Lab
- ABG
- Titration of drugs/therapies as ordered

Assess skin status
- Check incision lines, noting dimensions, drainage, appearance, presence of dressings, etc.
- Turn patient and check skin for burns, pressure areas, breaks in skin, bruises, edema
- Keep patient covered and warm slowly

Family should be allowed in as soon as patient becomes stable.

INTRA-AORTIC BALLOON THERAPY (IABP)

The intra-aortic balloon is most often inserted through the femoral artery into the descending aorta where displacement of blood by counterpulsation elicits physiological benefits. The balloon inflates and deflates in conjunction with events in the cardiac cycle. Inflation should occur during diastole when the aortic valve closes and increases the aortic pressure and improves coronary blood flow and perfusion. Deflation should occur at the onset of systole and lower the aortic pressure, ventricular resistance and decrease afterload. This increases cardiac output by approximately 10-20 percent and decreases myocardial oxygen demand.

Indications for use of counterpulsation
- Cardiogenic shock
- Weaning from cardiopulmonary bypass
- Mechanical complications of an acute myocardial infarction
- Papillary muscle rupture
- Ventricular septal defect

- Pre-infarction or post infarction unstable angina that is resistant to medical therapy
- Prophylactic support for severely ischemic myocardium during coronary angiography or anesthesia induction
- As a bridge to cardiac transplantation
- Valvular disease

Contraindications to IABP

- Aortic insufficiency
- Dissecting aortic or thoracic aneurysm
- Chronic end-stage heart disease
- Severe peripheral vascular disease
- Organic brain syndrome
- Irreversible brain damage
- Absent femoral pulses
- Recent trauma resulting in internal bleeding
- Active bleeding ulcer
- Blood dyscrasias
- Previous aortofemoral or aortoiliac bypass grafts

Complications

- Ruptured balloon
- Catheter fracture
- Occlusion of the left subclavian artery
- Obstruction of the subclavian, carotid, or renal arteries
- Diminished left radial pulse
- Sudden drop in urine output

- Flank pain
- Dizziness
- Decreased perfusion to feet
- Aortic intimal hematoma or dissection
- Thrombi on the balloon, the introducer sheath, or at the graft site

Hemodynamic Effects of IABP

- Decreased peak aortic systolic pressure
- Increased diastolic intra-aortic pressure
- Decreased arterial end diastolic pressure
- Decreased peak ventricular pressure
- Decreased LVEDP
- Increased CO/CI
- Decreased pulmonary capillary resistance

From Clinical Educational Services Information. Used by permission of Datascope Inc. Montvale, New Jersey

IABP TERMINOLOGY

Afterload—the amount of pressure against which the left ventricle must work during systole to open the aortic valve or the amount of wall tension created within the ventricle during the systolic phase of the cardiac cycle, measured by SVR or PVR

Assisted Aortic End-diastolic pressure (AOEDP)—the lowest diastolic pressure in the aortic which is affected by the deflation of the Intra-aortic balloon (IAB)

Assisted Systole (AS)—the systolic pressure which follows an assisted aortic end-diastolic pressure and should be lower than the unassisted systolic pressure

Atrial Systole—the contraction of the atria which causes an increase in the volume to the ventricles and is often referred to as atrial kick

Counterpulsation—the alternating inflation and deflation of the IABP during diastole and systole, respectively

Diastole—the relaxation of the heart muscle that begins when the aortic valve closes

Diastolic Augmentation—the resultant elevation of peak diastolic blood pressure due to the inflation of the IABP and the subsequent displacement of stroke volume

Dicrotic Notch—the area on an arterial pressure waveform that signifies aortic valve closure

Ejection Fraction—the percent of left ventricular end-diastolic volume which is ejected during systole (Normal 60-70%)

Isovolumetric Contraction—the phase in the mechanical cardiac cycle when all four valves are closed, causing no change in volume but causing a rapid increase in the ventricular pressure due to the ventricle attempting to overcome the unassisted end diastolic pressure; onset of systole and the phase where the majority of myocardial oxygen is consumed

Isovolumetric Relaxation—the phase in the mechanical cardiac cycle when all four valves are closed and there is no change in the ventricular volume but where there is a rapid decrease in pressure; onset of diastole

Mean Arterial Pressure (MAP)—the time-averaged pressure throughout each cycle of the heartbeat.

The ICU Quick Reference 337

Pacer Reject—the ability of the IABP to distinguish between an R wave and a pacer spike; the pacer spike is rejected and the R wave is used as the trigger event

Preload—the left ventricular end-diastolic volume and the amount of pressure it exerts on the walls of the left ventricle; assessed by the PCWP

Rapid Ventricular Ejection Phase—the period following the opening of the aortic valve where approximately 75% of the stroke volume is ejected from the left ventricle

Refractory Period—a 300 msec window after the R wave in which the IABP will not accept another trigger event; coincides with the segment and T wave

Safety Chamber—a closed gas, volume-limiting chamber that provides a "reverse" image of the action of the IAB

Stroke Volume—the amount of blood ejected by the left ventricle with each beat of the heart

Suprasystolic Augmentation—the diastolic augmentation that is greater than the systolic pressure

Systemic Vascular Resistance (SVR)—the resistance to ventricular ejection that is a measure of afterload

Systole—the phase of the cardiac cycle in which the heart is contracting

Threshold—the minimum voltage required by IABP to sense an EKG trigger

Timing— the inflation and deflation of the IABP in concert with the mechanical cardiac cycle

Trigger—the signal used by the IABP to identify the beginning of the next cardiac cycle and to deflate the IAB if it is not already deflated

Unassisted Aortic End-Diastolic Pressure—the aortic end diastolic pressure without IABP intervention

Unassisted Systole (UAS)—the systolic pressure which does not follow the deflation of the IAB

Ventricular Filling—the passive flow of blood from the atria into the ventricles

From Clinical Educational Services Information. Used by permission of Datascope Inc. Montvale, New Jersey

IABP WAVEFORM

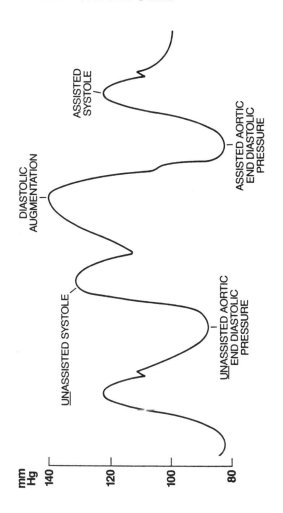

From Clinical Educational Services Information. Used by permission of Datascope Inc. Montvale, New Jersey

SYMPTOMS OF CARDIAC TAMPONADE

- Increased venous pressure (CVP over 12)
- Decreased blood pressure with narrowing pulse pressure
- Muffled or diminished heart sounds
- JVD with the head of the bed elevated 30-45 degrees
- Dyspnea
- Pulsus paradoxus (disappearance of pulse during inspiration)
- Cyanosis
- Decreased CO/CI
- Heart rate increased 20 beats/min or more from normal
- Equalization of CVP, PCWP, RA and LA pressures
- Abrupt cessation of previously heavy chest tube (mediastinal) drainage
- Increased SVR
- Cold, clammy skin
- Widening of mediastinum on X-ray
- Electrical alternans
- Enlarged cardiac silhouette on X-ray
- Decreased EKG voltage
- Apprehension, anxiety

CARDIAC CATHETERIZATION COMPLICATIONS

- Dysrhythmias (vasovagal problems, bradycardias, ventricular ectopy)
- Hemorrhage
- Allergic reactions to contrast media (hypotension, anaphylaxis)
- Renal failure
- Perforation of atria, ventricles, or arteries
- Embolism
- Damage to structures at insertion site
- Death (occurs in less than 1%)

PERCUTANEOUS TRANSLUMINAL CORONARY ANGIOPLASTY (PTCA) COMPLICATIONS

- Problems associated with cardiac catheterization
- Dissection of the coronary arteries
- Vasospasms involving the coronary arteries
- Dysrhythmias
- Intimal injury
- Sudden death

If chest pain occurs after PTCA, do not give morphine. Instead, use procardia and/or nitroglycerine.

CAUSES OF CORONARY ARTERY REOCCLUSION AFTER PTCA

Approximately ⅓ to ¼ will restenose in less than 1 year

- Thrombus that occludes the vessel
- False lumen (pseudoaneurysm)
- Air embolism
- Coronary artery spasm
- Plaque fragment embolus

WOLFF-PARKINSON-WHITE (WPW) SYNDROME

The impulse is conducted down an abnormal pathway (bundle of Kent) bypassing the AV node, while another impulse from a normal pathway (bundle of His) is concurrently conducted, so that the ventricle is stimulated from 2 directions.

- PR is < 0.12
- Slurred upstroke on R wave = delta wave
- Fused delta wave with RS of QRS with a fused complex usually > 0.12
- Type A has upright QRS, inverted T, and depressed ST in leads V1-V3
- Type B has downward QRS, upright T, and elevated ST in leads V1-V3
- Occurs most frequently in young adults
- Often associated with PSVT and atrial fibrillation
- Do not give digoxin—this will accentuate the problem. Recommended drug for WPW is procainamide 10 mg 1 kg over 5 min.

WELLEN'S SYNDROME
- Proximal LAD narrowing
- Usually admitted with unstable angina
- No Q waves
- No to minimal enzyme elevation
- Pain responds to nitroglycerin
- No to little abnormality
- Terminal T wave is negative
- Transient QT prolongation
- Negative U wave in the terminal part of the negative T
- Negative T waves in leads V2 and V3

RESPIRATORY CARE

TABLE OF CONTENTS

Oxygen Delivery Systems	347
Causes of Inadequate Alveolar Ventilation	347
Causes of Decreased Diffusion	348
Causes of Decreased Oxygen Transport	348
Pulmonary Terminology	349
Determining Problems With Ventilators	350
Hazards of Oxygen Therapy	351
Oxygen Toxicity	352
Formulas and Normals for Respiratory Equations	352
Indications for Mechanical Ventilation	354
Problems Associated With Mechanical Ventilation	355
Ventilator Modes	355
Peep	357
Guide to Initial Settings of Ventilators	359
Indications for Weaning From Ventilator	360
Determining ABG Results	361
Continuous Mixed Venous Oxygen Saturation Monitoring	362
Normals For Mixed Venous Blood Gases	363
Common Causes and Treatment for Acid Base Disorders	363
Breath Sounds	365
Oxygen Dissociation Curve	367
Comparison of Bronchitis Versus Emphysema	368
Ventilation Perfusion Scans	368
Adult Respiratory Distress Syndrome	369
ARDS Physiology	370

OXYGEN DELIVERY SYSTEMS

Nasal cannula	1-6 L/minute (each L/min = approximately 4% oxygen)
Simple mask	35-60%
Non-rebreathing mask	90-100%
Venturi mask	24-40%
Tracheal mask	35-70%
T-piece	25-70%
Room air	21%

CAUSES OF INADEQUATE ALVEOLAR VENTILATION

- Lack of or decreased pulmonary surfactant
- Abnormally high pCO_2 (above 45)
- Depression or damage to cerebral respiratory center (stroke, head injury, CNS depressant drugs)
- Paralysis of respiratory muscles (cord transection)
- Neuromuscular diseases (Guillain-Barré, myasthenia gravis, tetanus)
- Spinal cord injuries to C 1-5
- Asthma, bronchitis, COPD
- Restrictive lung diseases
- Morbid obesity (Pickwickian syndrome)
- Deformity of thoracic cage (kyphosis, scoliosis, pectus excavatum)
- Trauma to lung tissue, pneumo or hemothorax

CAUSES OF DECREASED DIFFUSION

- Removal of a portion of a membrane (lobectomy)
- Alteration of alveoli (atelectasis, COPD, pneumonia, pulmonary edema)
- Increase in thickness of respiratory membrane called alveolo-capillary block (pulmonary edema)
- Ventilation and perfusion mismatching
- Pulmonary infarct or embolism

CAUSES OF DECREASED OXYGEN TRANSPORT

- Anemia
- Hypovolemia
- Decreased cardiac output
- Carbon monoxide poisoning
- Vasoconstriction
- Hypotension
- Occlusions by thrombi
- Tissue ischemia

$\dot{V}$ = ventilation/minute

$\dot{Q}$ = perfusion of blood/minute

V/Q ratio = respiratory quotient, (normal 0.8)

$\dot{V}/\dot{Q}$ = index of oxygen transport in the lungs *(the difference between inspired tension and arterial tension per minute)*

If $\dot{V}/\dot{Q}$ is less than 0.8, there is a decrease of minute ventilation to perfusion, creating a physiologic shunt *(hypoxemia, atelectasis and pneumonia)*

If $\dot{V}/Q$ is greater than 0.8, there is normal ventilation but a decrease in perfusion, which increases dead space and wastes ventilation *(pulmonary emboli and shock)*

PULMONARY TERMINOLOGY

- **Rate (f)**: Breaths/minute, normal 12-20; above 30 takes lots of energy; above 40 leads to fatigue and respiratory failure; increases oxygen need
- **Tidal Volume (V_T)**: Volume in one normal breath either inhaled or exhaled; normal 5-8 cc/kg ideal body weight, dead space is approximately 150 cc or 30% of tidal volume, for sighs never put more than 15 cc/kg ideal body weight
- **Minute Volume or Minute Ventilation ($\dot{V}E$)**: $VE = V_T \times f$; normal 5-10 L/min; septic shock patients have 15 or more L/minute; less than 5 L/min or more than 10L/min probably won't wean from ventilator
- **Vital Capacity (VC)**: The maximum volume of air exhaled after a maximum inspiration; Use nomogram of predicted values, but usually can be approximated at 65 cc/kg body weight; if VC is low, patient cannot cough or move excretions
- **Maximum Inspiratory Pressure (MIP) Negative Inspiratory Force (NIF)**: How much negative pressure can be generated: (normal -80 to -100) if patient cannot generate at least -20, he cannot maintain airway independently and breathe
- **Inspiratory Capacity (IC)**: Volume of gas inhaled from an end tidal exhalation
- **Forced Vital Capacity (FVC)**: Pulmonary function test: Inhale fully and exhale as quickly and forcefully as possible until all air has been exhaled
- **Forced Expiratory Volume in one second (FEV_1)** FEV_1/VC%: normal in adults > 75%
- **Residual Volume (RV)**: the volume of air that remains in the lungs at the end of a maximum exhalation

- **Inspiratory Reserve Volume (IRV):** the maximum volume of air that can be inhaled after a tidal breath has been taken
- **Expiratory Reserve Volume (ERV):** the maximum volume of air that can be exhaled after the end of normal expiration
- **Total Lung Capacity (TLC)** = V_T+ IRV+ ERV+ RV
- **Vital Capacity (VC)** = V_T+ IRV + ERV
- **Inspiratory Capacity (IC)** = V_T + IRV
- **Functional Residual Capacity (FRC)** = ERV + RV

From Beth Minssen, R.N., M.A. C.C.R.N. *Mechanical Ventilation*, 2nd. ed. 1990. Panhandle Education for Nurses, Lubbock, Texas. Used by permission of the author.

DETERMINING PROBLEMS WITH VENTILATOR USING PEAK INSPIRATORY PRESSURE (PIP) AND PLATEAU PRESSURES

- PIP, Plateau unchanged—normal
- PIP increased, plateau unchanged or slightly increased
  - Mucous plug
  - Bronchospasm
- PIP and plateau unchanged but PCWP (pulmonary capillary wedge pressure) decreased, PAP (pulmonary artery pressure) increased, CVP (central venous pressure) increased, CO/CI (cardiac output/cardiac index) decreased, (SVR) Systemic vascular resistance increased, cyanosis and JVD (jugular vein distention) present:
  - Pulmonary embolus
  - Tension pneumothorax
  - Cardiac tamponade
  - Dissecting aneurysm
- PIP, Plateau increased:
  - Tension pneumothorax (with sudden onset)

- Atelectasis
- Pneumonia
- ARDS

From Beth Minssen, R.N., M.A. C.C.R.N. Mechanical Ventilation, 2nd. ed. 1990. Panhandle Education for Nurses, Lubbock, Texas. Used by permission of the author.

HAZARDS OF OXYGEN THERAPY

1. Oxygen induced bradypnea
2. Absorption atelectasis
3. Oxygen toxicity
   - FIO_2 (fraction of inspired O_2) above 60% for more than 48 hours; or 100% FIO_2 after 6 hours can produce pulmonary changes in adults
   - Decrease in tracheal mucus flow
   - Decreased macrophage activity
   - Decreased vital capacity
   - Endothelial cell damage and increased lung water
   - Progressive atelectasis
   - Decreased surfactant production
   - Decreased compliance
   - Increased A-a gradient
   - Decreased diffusing capacity
   - Decreased pulmonary capillary blood volume
   - Capillary injury
   - Platelet aggregation

From Beth Minssen, R.N., M.A. C.C.R.N. Mechanical Ventilation, 2nd. ed. 1990. Panhandle Education for Nurses, Lubbock, Texas. Used by permission of the author.

OXYGEN TOXICITY

Early Signs	Late Signs
Restlessness	Severe dyspnea
Fatigue	Respiratory distress
Malaise	Cyanosis
Dyspnea	Asphyxia
Coughing	Nausea/vomiting
Anorexia	Peripheral paresthesias
Retrosternal discomfort	Hypoxemia

FORMULAS AND NORMALS FOR RESPIRATORY EQUATIONS

Arterial Oxygen Content (CaO_2)

$$CaO_2 = Hgb \times 1.34 \times \% \text{ saturation}$$

Normal: 20 cc/100 cc   panic level = less than 11

$$CaO_2 = O_2 \text{ capacity} \times O_2 \text{ saturation} + (0.0031 \times PaO_2)$$

Oxygen Transport = O_2 delivery = DO_2

$$DO_2 = H_2O \text{ content} \times 10 \times \text{Cardiac output}$$

Normal: 1000-1200 cc/minute

$$O_2 \text{ capacity} = Hgb \times 1.34$$

$$O_2 \text{ saturation} = \frac{CaO_2}{O_2 \text{ capacity}} \times 100$$

Compliance (Cl)

$$Cl = \text{Change in Volume/Change in Pressure}$$

NOTE changes in trends!

$$\text{Oxygen Consumption} = CO \times Hgb \times 13.9 \, (SaO_2 - S_vO_2)$$

Normal: 250 cc/min

P50—the partial pressure of oxygen at which Hgb is 50% saturated

Normal: 26.6 mm Hg

Static Compliance (Cst)

$$Cst = \frac{V_T}{\text{Plateau Pressure–PEEP}}$$

Normal: 35-50 cc/cm H_2O

Dynamic Compliance (Cdyn)

$$Cdyn = \frac{V_T}{\text{PIP–PEEP}}$$

A-a Gradient (Alveolar—Arterial Oxygen Gradient)

$$\text{A-a gradients} = PAO_2 - PaO_2$$

$$PAO_2 = [(760-47) \times FIO_2] - \frac{PaCO_2}{0.8}$$

$$PAO_2 = (\text{Barometric pressure} - \text{vapor pressure of } H_2O) \times FIO_2 - \frac{(PaCO_2)}{0.8}$$

Normal: 10-16 depending on age and FIO_2

Shunting

- **True shunt**—the venous blood that does not participate in gas exchange
- **Calculated shunt**—based on the patient being on 100% O_2 for at least 15 minutes

$$\frac{Qs}{Qt} = \frac{(PaO_2 - PaO_2) \times 0.003}{(CaO_2 - CvO_2) + (PaO_2 - PaO_2)(0.003)} \times 100$$

- Qs = shunted portion of cardiac output

- Qt = total cardiac output
- 0.003 = amount of oxygen in 100 cc plasma
- PAO_2 = partial pressure of alveolar oxygen
- PaO_2 = Partial pressure of arterial oxygen
- CaO_2 = arterial oxygen content
- CvO_2 = venous oxygen content
- Normal physiologic shunt = 2-5% of cardiac output or 5 ml/dl
- For every 15 on A-a gradient, there is a 1% shunt

From Beth Minssen, R.N., M.A. C.C.R.N. Mechanical Ventilation, 2nd. ed. 1990. Panhandle Education for Nurses, Lubbock, Texas. Used by permission of the author.

INDICATIONS FOR MECHANICAL VENTILATION

Refractory hypoxemia

- Pulmonary edema
    - Cardiogenic
    - Non-cardiogenic (ARDS)
- Pneumonia
- Pulmonary embolism

Hypercapnia

- COPD
- Hypoventilation
    - Post anesthesia
    - Drugs
    - Overdose
    - CVA
    - ALS

- Cardiac arrest

PROBLEMS ASSOCIATED WITH MECHANICAL VENTILATION
- Right bronchus intubation
- Barotrauma
- Alveolar hyperventilation or hypoventilation
- Pulmonary artery pressures increase
- Decreased venous return
- Vena cava compression
- Decreased cardiac output
- Decreased blood pressure
- Nutrition deficiencies
- Communication problems
- Psychological problems
- GI complications (*ileus, stress ulcer*)
- Atelectasis
- Tracheal necrosis (*cuff pressure should be kept below 25 cm H_2O or 20 mm Hg to avoid this*)
- Cuff leak

VENTILATOR MODES

CMV *Controlled Mechanical Ventilation-*
Ventilator delivers a set number of breaths per minute of a set tidal volume; used for apneic patients only.

AC *Assist Control*
Ventilator delivers a set number of breaths per minute of a set tidal volume, but breaths may be triggered by patient effort, and each breath will be of the set tidal volume; usually requires set

or manually given signs since each breath has the preset volume; useful when patient respirations are rapid and with inadequate volume.

IMV *Intermittent Mandatory Ventilation*
Ventilator delivers a set number of breaths per minute at a set tidal volume, but the patient is able to breathe spontaneously with his own tidal volume; the problem with this setting is that the machine does not take into consideration that the patient may be in the middle of a breath when the preset breath is delivered.

SIMV *Synchronized Intermittent Mandatory Ventilation*
Basically the same as IMV except that the ventilator delivers breaths in synchronization with the patient's spontaneous effort; most ventilators these days have only this setting rather than IMV.

PSV *Pressure Support Ventilation*
Ventilator delivers a set amount of positive pressure to supplement the patient's spontaneous respirations and decreases the work of breathing; used to decrease patient's effort and labor of breathing and when attempting to wean patients off ventilation. It must be used on spontaneously breathing patients.

PEEP *Positive End Expiratory Pressure*
Ventilator applies a set amount of positive pressure above that of atmospheric pressure at the end of the inspiration cycle; this keeps the alveoli from completely collapsing and causing a larger amount of inspiratory pressure to be necessary to reopen the alveoli; this also causes

an increase in the amount of surface to oxygenate: used when increasing the percentage of oxygen is unable to oxygenate the patient to an adequate level.

CPAP *Continuous Positive Airway Pressure*

Similar to PEEP, but is used with spontaneously breathing patients; the patient may be on the ventilator but the ventilator is not delivering any breaths; the patient is exhaling against positive airway pressures and this improves oxygen tension and can facilitate lower percentages of oxygen being used; used with weaning PEEP-dependent patients.

PEEP

Positive End Expiratory Pressure (PEEP) is the application of positive pressure to keep alveoli from collapsing. The goal is to enhance tissue oxygenation and maintain adequate PaO_2 without utilizing high FIO_2 while still sustaining cardiovascular function

- Low or physiologic PEEP = 1 to 5 cm H_2O
- Moderate PEEP = 5 to 20 cm H_2O
- High PEEP = above 20 cm H_2O

Optimum PEEP = maximum benefits (increased oxygen transport, increased FRC, increased compliance, increased PaO_2, decreased shunt) without negative cardiopulmonary effects (decreased venous return, decreased cardiac output, decreased BP, increased shunt, increased dead space, barotrauma) at safe levels of FIO_2.

Indications for use of PEEP

- Refractory hypoxemia (ARDS, pulmonary infiltrates)

- Systemic injury with diffuse metabolic lung injury
- PaO_2 less than 60 on FIO_2 greater than 70%
- A-a gradient greater than 300 on FIO_2 of 100%
- Shunt greater than 30
- Recurrent atelectasis with low FRC
- Reduced compliance

Contraindications for use of PEEP
- Hypovolemia
- Untreated pneumothorax
- Increased ICP
- COPD
- Severe cardiac impairment

Side Effects from PEEP:
- Decreased CO/CI, decreased BP
- Barotrauma
    - Pneumothorax
    - Pneumomediastinum
    - Subcutaneous emphysema
- Decreased O_2 delivery
- Decreased urinary output

Initiating PEEP
Before beginning obtain baseline values of ABG, CO, CI, PCWP, PAP, PVR, PVO_2, SVO_2, BP, HR, breath sounds, plateau pressure, PIP, f (respiratory rate), VT, VE, compliance, CaO_2, A-a gradient, SaO_2, and patient appearance/assessment

Start at 5 cm H_2O and increase with 2 to 5 cm H_2O every 30 min if necessary. If necessary evaluation after 30 mins.

From Beth Minssen, R.N., M.A. C.C.R.N. *Mechanical Ventilation*, 2nd. ed. 1990., Panhandle Education for Nurses, Lubbock, Texas. Used by permission of the author.

GUIDE TO INITIAL SETTINGS OF VENTILATORS

- V_T—5 to 8 cc/kg of ideal body weight, plus sighs of 10 to 15 cc/kg
- Sigh volume and rate—1 ½ to 2 times V_T every 5 minutes; not used with increased V_T, PEEP, or pressure cycled ventilators
- Flow rate—set for approximate I:E ratio, rate and V_T, and flow rate; greater than 40 L/minute decreases inspiratory time and causes increased pressure:

$$\frac{V_T}{I} = cc/sec$$

$$(cc/sec \div 1000) \times 60 = L/min$$

Example:

$V_T = 500$ Rate = 10 I:E ratio = 1:2

$\dfrac{60 \text{ sec}}{10 \text{ rate}} = 6$ sec resp cycle $\dfrac{6 \text{ sec}}{3 \text{ sec}} = 2$ sec   6 sec resp cycle = I 2 sec E 4 sec

$\dfrac{500 \text{ cc}}{2 \text{ sec}} = 250$ cc/sec   = 0.25 L/sec × 60 sec
= 15 L/minute

What flow rate would be needed if rate increased to 14?

$\dfrac{60 \text{ sec}}{14 \text{ rate}} = 4.28$ sec $\dfrac{4.28}{1 + 2} = 1.43$ $\dfrac{500}{1.43} = 349$

$0.349 \times 60 = 21$ L/min

- * Pressure limit—Set at 20 cm above PIP of normal breath
- * FIO$_2$—start at 50%, unless pt is status post cardiac arrest; then begin at 100%. Obtain ABGs after 15-30 min, and reduce per the following equation:

$$\frac{PaO_2 - 100}{7} = \text{percentage of FIO}_2 \text{ by which you can decrease}$$

Example: On 100%, ABG PaO$_2$ of 215,
$$\frac{215 - 100}{7} = 16$$
Therefore the FIO$_2$ can be reduced to 84-85%

- * Sensitivity—set at -2 cm H$_2$O
- * Rate—10-15 per minute
- * Humidifier—35 to 37 degrees centigrade

From Beth Minssen, R.N., M.A. C.C.R.N. Mechanical Ventilation, 2nd. ed. 1990., Panhandle Education for Nurses, Lubbock, Texas. Used by permission of the author.

INDICATIONS FOR WEANING FROM VENTILATOR

- Adequate hemoglobin, oxygen content and oxygen transport
- Acid-base balance, A-a gradient acceptable
- No fever
- No electrolyte imbalance
- No sign/symptoms of inspiratory muscle fatigue (check inspiratory rate, V$_T$, depth pattern, muscles of respiration)
- Adequate nutrition avoiding carbohydrate loading—ideally 50% of calories should be fat
- Cardiovascular stability (adequate BP, little to no dysrhythmias)
- Awake and alert

- Rested, with no suppressant drugs (don't try to wean at night or with activities)
- Spontaneous respirations with a negative inspiratory force of - 20 at least; - 50 is best
- PaO_2 above 60 on FIO_2 below 50% and maximum PEEP 5 cm H_2O
- Vital capacity equal to or above 10 to 15 cc/kg ideal weight
- Resting minute ventilation less than 10 L/min and maintain $PaCO_2$ below 40 (normal 65-75 cc/kg)
- Tidal volume equal to or above 5 cc/kg
- Reversal or stabilization *of underlying disease process*

From Beth Minssen, R.N., M.A. C.C.R.N. Mechanical Ventilation, 2nd. ed. 1990., Panhandle Education for Nurses, Lubbock, Texas. Used by permission of the author.

DETERMINING ABG RESULTS
(at sea level) [in higher altitudes, PO_2 and SaO_2 are lower]

pH	7.40	Normal
	7.39-7.35	Compensate acidosis
	≤ 7.34	Acidosis
	7.41-7.45	Compensated alkalosis
	≥ 7.46	Alkalosis
pCO_2	40	Normal
	35-39	Compensated
	< 35	Uncompensated
	41- 45	Compensated
	> 45	Uncompensated

pO$_2$ 80-100 Normal
(lower in newborn and elderly)
(80-1 for every year over 60)

- Determine acidity or alkalinity using pH
- Determine metabolic or respiratory component as follows using CO$_2$ result:
  - Metabolic
    - Low CO$_2$ with acidosis
    - High CO$_2$ with alkalosis
  - Respiratory
    - Low CO$_2$ with alkalosis
    - High CO$_2$ with acidosis

Respiratory Insufficiency = PCO$_2$ above 50 and/or PO$_2$ below 60

CONTINUOUS MIXED VENOUS OXYGEN SATURATION (SVO$_2$) MONITORING

- Performed with a fiberoptic oximetry pulmonary artery catheter that is connected with a monitor that gives a continuous digital display of the percentage of mixed venous oxygen saturation.
- The fiberoptic carries red and infrared light from the monitor to the distal tip of the catheter. The light that emanates from this fiber scatters off of the red blood cells that are flowing past the tip, and the backscattered light is received by another fiber. The SvO$_2$ measurement is derived from the analyzing of the intensities of the light.
- SvO$_2$ monitoring often provides the first early warning signs that the patient's oxygenation status is deteriorating. Changes occur quickly and are present prior to arterial compromise.

- Normal SvO_2 is 75% [SvO_2 < 60%—cardiac decompensation].
- Normal PvO_2 is 40 mm Hg.
- AV difference = SaO_2-SvO_2; normal is 20-30.
- AV oxygen content difference = CaO_2-CvO_2 ; normal is 4.5-6 ml/dl.

NORMALS FOR MIXED VENOUS BLOOD GASES

pH	=	7.36
pO_2	=	35-40
pCO_2	=	41-51
$SvO2$	=	70-75%
$HCO3$	=	22-26

COMMON CAUSES AND TREATMENT FOR ACID BASE DISORDERS

Metabolic Acidosis

  Causes
- Diamox therapy
- Ketoacidosis (diabetic or alcoholic ketoacidosis, starvation ketosis)
- Lactic acidosis (inadequate circulation or drug therapy)
- Poisoning
- Renal failure

Treatment
- Treat underlying cause
- Sodium bicarbonate if necessary

Metabolic Alkalosis
Causes
- Chloride depletion (vomiting, gastric suctioning, or diuretic therapy except with Diamox)
- Excessive sodium bicarbonate administration
- Hyperadrenocorticism
- Severe potassium depletion

Treatment
- Treat underlying cause; Diamox (excretes bicarbonation)
- Potassium chloride (if renal function adequate)

Respiratory Acidosis
Causes
- Cardiopulmonary failure
- Chronic obstructive lung disease
- Hypoventilation
- Neuromuscular disorders
- Respiratory center depression (cerebral disorder or drug therapy)

Treatment
- Increase respiratory rate
- Increase VT

Respiratory Alkalosis
Causes
- Brain-stem disease
- Cirrhosis
- Fever
- Hypoxia
- Overventilation by a mechanical ventilator

- Psychogenic hyperventilation
- Pulmonary embolism
- Salicylate overdose
- Thyrotoxicosis
- Pain

Treatment
- Decrease respiratory rate
- Sedation
- Decrease V_T
- Analgesics

BREATH SOUNDS

Normal Sounds
Bronchial
Normally heard from larynx to the top of the sternum; abnormal if heard anywhere else and may mean patient has a consolidation:
- Harsh sounds like air blowing through a long tube
- Also known as tubular breath sounds
- Inspiration/expiration ratio is 1:2 with a pause between inspiration and expiration

Vesicular
Normally heard over most of the lung tissues:
- Soft, swishing-type sounds, rustling
- Inspiration/expiration ratio is 2:1 with no pause between inspiration and expiration

Bronchovesicular
Normally heard in right lung apex and to each side of the sternum, they are abnormal if heard anywhere else:

- Mixture of both bronchial and vesicular sounds
- Inspiration = expiration with no pause between

Adventitious Breath Sounds

Crackles *(also known as rales)* caused by fluid in the alveoli or airways; usually heard at the end of the inspiratory cycle

- *Fine crackles* sound like rubbing hairs between fingers near ear.
- *Medium crackles* sound like listening to a freshly opened can of soda.
- *Coarse crackles* sound like the rustling of cellophane.

Moist wheezes or gurgles *(also known as rhonchi)* are continuous sounds made as air passes through edematous or spasmodic airways, or through airways that are partially filled with mucous. They are usually heard during expiration even though they are continuous sounds.

- **Sibilant wheezes** sound high pitched and have a musical quality.
- **Sonorous wheezes** sound like a person snoring. These wheezes are caused by air passing through passageways that have a decreased lumen; they can be heard during expiration or inspiration.

Pleural friction rub is caused by inflammation of the pleura as they rub against each other; it sounds like rubbing leather together and stops if the patient holds his breath.

Voice Sounds

Bronchophony, if heard, probably indicates a pulmonary consolidation. Bronchophony is present if, when a patient repeats something such as "99", tones are less muffled and "99" can be clearly understood while auscultating lungs.

Egophony, if heard, probably indicates a pleural effusion or lung consolidation. Egophony is present if, when a patient says "e", it comes out sounding like "a" while lungs are auscultated.

Pectoriloquy is present if whispered words are clearly distinguished while auscultating lungs.

OXYGEN DISSOCIATION CURVE

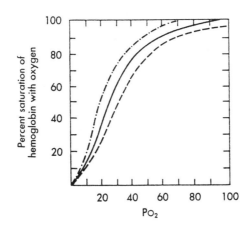

SHIFT TO THE LEFT	SHIFT TO THE RIGHT
Decreased temperature (hypothermia)	Increased temperature (hyperthermia)
Decreased acidity (alkalosis)	Increased acidity (acidosis)
Decreased CO_2 (hypocarbia)	Increased CO_2 (hypercarbia)
Decreased 2, 3 DPG	Increased 2, 3 DPG

COMPARISON OF BRONCHITIS VERSUS EMPHYSEMA

BRONCHITIS	EMPHYSEMA
"Blue Bloaters"	"Pink Puffers"
Cyanosis present	NO cyanosis
Mild to moderate SOB	Severe SOB
Cough present and productive	No cough
Mild to moderate CO_2 retention	No CO_2 retention until end stage
Mild to moderate hypoxemia	No hypoxemia until end stage
Weight stable	Weight loss cachexia
Improvement with bronchodilator	No improvement with bronchodialtors
COR Pulmonale	Barrel chest with hypertrophic accessory muscles of respiration

VENTILATION PERFUSION SCANS

Probability of Pulmonary Embolus	Defects
Normal, no pulmonary embolus	No perfusion defects
Low, (10% or less)	Small (involving less than 25% of lung segment) ventilation/perfusion mismatch. Ventilation/perfusion defects without X-ray changes. Perfusion

	defect smaller than X-ray density.
Intermediate (30-60%)	Perfusion defects with severe diffuse obstruction to lung. Perfusion defects the same size as X-ray densities. Single defect involving 25-90% of lung segment or large (greater than 90% of lung segment involved) defect.
High (greater than 90%)	2 or more medium (25-90% involved) or large (greater than 90% involved) perfusion defects. Perfusion defects larger than X-ray densities.

ADULT RESPIRATORY DISTRESS SYNDROME (ARDS)

- Hypoperfusion of the lungs
- Acute respiratory failure without airway obstruction and/or left ventricular failure
- Also known as shock lung, wet lung, Da Nang lung, or capillary leak syndrome

Causes

- Anaphylaxis
- Aspiration pneumonia
- DIC
- Fat embolus
- Multiple transfusions
- AIDS
- Amniotic embolus
- Drugs (heroin, methadone)
- Multi-system organ failure
- Oxygen toxicity

- Pancreatitis
- Sepsis
- Smoke inhalation

Signs and Symptoms
- Tachypnea
- Cyanosis
- Large A-a gradient
- Decreased functional residual capacity (FRC)
- Hypoxia even with 100% oxygen and high ventilation pressures (up to 80 cm H_2O)

- Prolonged coronary artery bypass
- Shock
- Trauma

- Dyspnea
- Tachycardia
- Decreased lung compliance
- Diffuse interstitial pattern on X-ray (after 12-24 hrs)
- Crackles/wheezes may or may not be present

ARDS PHYSIOLOGY

- Hypoperfusion
- Increased complement system
- Histamine release
- Decreased fibronectin
- Capillary leakage
- Decreased surfactant
- Decreased FRC
- Atelectasis
- Acidosis

- Hypoxia
- Platelet aggregation
- Oxygen radicals released
- Increased capillary permeability
- Interstitial and intra-alveolar edema
- Decreased lung compliance
- V/Q mismatching
- Hypoxemia
- Death

RENAL AND ENDOCRINE SYSTEMS

TABLE OF CONTENTS

Electrolyte and Mineral Imbalances/Causes 373
Daily Approximate Requirements 376
Common Signs and Symptoms of Endocrine
Dysfunction 376
The Renin-Angiotensin Aldosterone Feedback
System 379
Fluid and Electrolyte Imbalances 380
Endocrine System Glands and Hormones Secreted . . 388
Endocrine Problems 389
Syndrome of Inappropriate Antidiuretic
Hormone 392
Differences Between Prerenal, Renal,
and Postrenal Failure 394
Glomerular Filtration Rate 395

ELECTROLYTE AND MINERAL IMBALANCES/CAUSES

Hypoglycemia *(< 60 mg/dl)*
  Causes: Prolonged stress, inadequate glucose, adrenal insufficiency, insulinoma, hypothyroidism, liver disease, MAO inhibitors

Hyperglycemia *(>130 mg/dl)*
  Causes: Sepsis, hypothermia, infections, surgery, trauma, stress, DKA, pheochromocytoma, hyperthyroidism, diuretics

Hypocalcemia *(< 8.5 mg/dl)*
  Causes: Stress, blood administration, renal failure, poor calcium intake, diarrhea, Vitamin D deficiency, Cushing's syndrome, hypoparathyroidism, magnesium depletion, high fat diet, gastrectomy, bone metastasis, pancreatitis, hyperphosphatemia, phenytoin, phenobarbital, alkalosis, decreased serum albumin

Hypercalcemia *(> 10.5 mg/dl)*
  Causes: Hyperparathyroidism, thyrotoxicosis, immobilization, hypophosphatemia, Vitamin D intoxication, acidosis (increased level of ionized CA^{++}), chronic use of thiazide diuretics, large dietary intake of calcium, multiple myeloma, metastatic carcinoma, Addison's disease, renal failure

Hypokalemia (< 3.5 mEq/L)
Causes: Diuresis, decreased potassium intake, alkalosis, Fanconi's syndrome, renal tubular acidosis, liver disease, diuretic use, laxative abuse, nasogastric suction or drainage, diarrhea, excess aldosterone secretion, vomiting, starvation, trauma, excessive licorice ingestion

Hyperkalemia (> 5.0 mEq/L)
Causes: Increased intake of potassium, renal disease, decreased cardiac output, sodium depletion, aldosterone insufficiency, burns, trauma, rhabdomyolysis, acidosis, tissue catabolism, malignant hyperthermia, Addison's disease, ibuprofen, indomethacin

Hypernatremia (>145 mEq/L)
Causes: Water loss in excess of sodium loss, diabetes insipidus, potassium depletion, hypercalcemia, increased sodium bicarbonate or sodium chloride use, laxative abuse, uncontrolled diabetes mellitus, renal tubular disease, osmotic diuresis, dehydration, Cushing's syndrome, burns, steroids, carbenicillin

Hyponatremia with hypovolemia (< 135 mEq/L)
Causes: Infection, nausea, vomiting, diarrhea, hyperglycemia, malnutrition, diuretics, trauma, diaphoresis, nasogastric suction or drainage, Addison's disease, chronic renal insufficiency

Hyponatremia with normal or excess volume (< 135 mEq/L)
Causes: Congestive heart failure, cirrhosis, Syndrome of Inappropriate Anti-diuretic Hormone (SIADH), psychogenic polydypsia

Hypophosphatemia (< 3.0 mg/L)
Causes: Hyperventilation, chronic alcoholism, hyperparathyroidism, parenteral hyperalimentation, malabsorption syndrome, rickets, antacid abuse, Fanconi's syndrome, hypomagnesemia, hypokalemia, glycosuria, thiazide diuretics

Hyperphosphatemia (> 4.5 mg/dl)
Causes: Hypoparathyroidism, laxative abuse, renal failure, cytotoxic drugs, excess phosphate PO or IV, Vitamin D excess, respiratory acidosis, neoplastic disease, tissue catabolism, rhabdomyolysis, thyrotoxicosis

Hypermagnesemia (> 2.5 mEq/L)
Causes: Acidosis, adrenal insufficiency, renal failure, excessive laxative or antacid use, increased magnesium intake

Hypomagnesemia (<1.5 mEq/L)
Causes: Starvation, parenteral hyperalimentation, excessive diuretic therapy, nasogastric suctioning or drainage, malabsorption syndrome, diarrhea, vomiting, alcoholism, hypocalcemia, hypoparathyroidism, hyperaldosteronism, DKA, hyperthyroidism, pancreatitis, colitis, cisplatin cancer treatment, amphotericin, tobramycin, gentamicin, digoxin, alkalosis (occasionally)

DAILY APPROXIMATE REQUIREMENTS

Sodium   3-4 mEq/kg/24 hours   60-150 mEq/24h

Potassium 2-3 mEq/kg/24 hours   40-240 mEq/24h

Calcium   50-100 mg/kg/24 hours 5-30 mEq/24h

Magnesium 0.4-0.9 mEq/kg/24 hours 10-45 mEq/24h

COMMON SIGNS AND SYMPTOMS OF ENDOCRINE DYSFUNCTION

Sign or symptom: *Weakness, fatigue, lethargy*

Possible Cause:
Addison's disease, Cushing's syndrome, adrenal crisis hypothyroidism, hyperparathyroidism, diabetes mellitus, hypoglycemia, pheochromocytoma, systemic lupus erythematosus, uremic syndrome, SIADH, HHNC, hypoglycemia

Sign or symptom: *Weight loss*

Possible Cause:
Hyperthyroidism, pheochromocytoma, Addison's disease, hyperparathyroidism, lupus erythematosus, uremic syndrome, diabetes insipidus, DKA

Sign or symptom: *Weight gain*

Possible Cause:
Cushing's syndrome, hypothyroidism, Type II diabetes mellitus, pituitary tumor, SIADH (**Note:** primary endocrine disorders account for less than 5% of obesity

cases where body weight is 30% or more above ideal; obesity may cause secondary endocrine and metabolic changes.)

Sign or symptom: *Body temperature changes*

Possible Cause:

Elevation: Thyrotoxicosis (thyroid storm), primary hypothalamic disease (after pituitary surgery)

Decreases: Addison's disease, hypoglycemia, myxedema coma

Sign or symptom: *Skin changes*

Possible Cause:

Hyperpigmentation: Addison's disease, post-op bilateral adrenalectomy for Cushing's disease, ACTH-producing pituitary tumor

Hirsutism: Cushing's syndrome, adrenal tumor, acromegaly

Coarse, dry skin: Myxedema, hypoparathyroidism, acromegaly, renal failure, DKA

Excessive sweating: Thyrotoxicosis, acromegaly, pheochromocytoma, hypoglycemia

Color changes: Uremic syndrome

Sign or symptom: *Anorexia*

Possible Cause:

Hyperparathyroidism, Addison's disease, DKA, hypothyroidism, SIADH, adrenal crisis

Sign or symptom: *Abdominal pain*
Possible Cause:
DKA, myxedema, Addisonian crisis, thyroid storm (thyrotoxicosis), adrenal crisis, hypoparathyroidism, pheochromocytoma

Sign or symptom: *Anemia*
Possible Cause:
Hypothyroidism, hypopituitarism, adrenal insufficiency, Cushing's disease, hyperparathyroidism, renal failure

Sign or symptom: *Bradycardia*
Possible Cause:
Myxedema coma

Sign or symptom: *Tachycardia*
Possible Cause:
Thyroid Storm or thyrotoxicosis, pheochromocytoma, uremic syndrome, DKA, HHNC, hypoglycemia, adrenal crisis, diabetes insipidus

Sign or symptom: *Hypertension*
Possible Cause:
Primary aldosteronism, pheochromocytoma, Cushing's syndrome, intrarenal failure

Sign or symptom: *Hypotension*
Possible Cause:
Myxedema coma, uremic syndrome, pre-renal failure, DKA, HHNC, adrenal crisis, diabetes insipidus

Sign or symptom: *Libido changes, sexual dysfunction*
Possible Cause:
Adrenal crisis, diabetes mellitus, hypopituitarism, gonadal failure, uremic syndrome, thyrotoxicosis, myxedema coma

THE RENIN-ANGIOTENSIN ALDOSTERONE FEEDBACK SYSTEM

- Decreased mean arterial pressure
- Decreased extracellular fluid volume
- Decreased serum sodium
- Juxtaglomerular cells secrete renin
- Renin converts angiotensinogen to angiotensin I
- Pulmonary enzyme converts angiotensin I to angiotensin II
- Angiotensin II constricts arterioles, increases blood pressure and stimulates adrenal cortex to release aldosterone
- Aldosterone increases sodium and water retention, which increases extracellular fluid volume and inhibits renin secretion

FLUID AND ELECTROLYTE IMBALANCES

HYPONATREMIA *(sodium below 135 mEq/L)*
- Headache
- Apathy
- Nausea
- Diarrhea
- Anxiety
- Anorexia
- Vomiting

HYPONATREMIA *with dehydration*
- Headache
- Apathy
- Nausea
- Diarrhea
- Sense of impending doom
- Stupor
- Weakness
- Muscle twitching
- Oliguria
- Hypotension
- Finger print edema to sternum (BAD sign)
- Anxiety
- Anorexia
- Vomiting
- Apprehension
- Confusion
- Dry mucous membranes
- Abdominal cramping
- Convulsions
- Anuria
- Tachycardia

HYPONATREMIA *with water retention*
- Confusion
- Weakness
- Coma → death
- Headache
- Convulsions

Treatment

- Restrict fluids
- Monitor I&O
- Hypertonic saline IV slowly

HYPERNATREMIA *(sodium above 145 mEq/L)*

- Hypertension *(with fluid retention)*
- Agitation
- Shortness of breath *(severe imbalance)*
- Manic behavior
- Death
- Irritability
- Seizures
- Dry mucous membranes
- Flushed skin
- Low-grade fever
- Intense thirst
- Tachycardia

- Hypotension *(without fluid retention)*
- Restlessness
- Convulsions *(severe imbalances)*
- Coma
- Lethargy
- Tremors
- Coma
- Rough, dry tongue
- Firm rubbery skin turgor
- Oliguria
- Some cardiac depression
- Increased cardiac output

Treatment

- Monitor cardiopulmonary status
- Monitor I&O
- Monitor urine and plasma osmolality

HYPOKALEMIA *(potassium below 3.5 mEq/L)*

- Dysrhythmias *(usually atrial unless hypokalemia is severe)*,
- Depressed ST segment or T wave inversion on EKG
- Muscle weakness
- Leg cramps
- Irritability
- Shallow respirations
- Enhanced effectiveness of digitalis *(to the point of toxicity)*
- Presence of prominent U wave
- Fatigue
- Drowsiness
- Coma
- Respiratory distress or arrest

Treatment

- Monitor cardiac rhythm
- Monitor I&O
- Monitor serum K level
- Potassium supplement PO or IV *(no faster than 10 mEq/hr IV through peripheral line)*

HYPERKALEMIA *(potassium above 5.0 mEq/L)*

- Bradycardia, lethal dysrhythmias, cardiac arrest, presence of peaked T wave and narrow QRS complex on EKG with levels up to 7.5 mEq/L, progressing to widened QRS complex, and then flattened P wave
- Prolonged PR interval and ST depression with levels up to 9 mEq/L

- P waves disappear and intraventricular conduction defects occur with levels > 9 mEq/L
- Progress to VF and death
- Apathy
- Areflexia
- Muscle weakness
- Abdominal cramping
- Diarrhea
- Confusion
- Numbness to extremities
- Flaccidity
- Nausea
- Oliguria

Treatment
- Levels up to 6.5 mEq/L sorbitol and sodium polystyrene sulfate
- Levels > 6.5 mEq/L glucose, insulin, sodium bicarbonate
- Levels > 7.5 mEq/L calcium gluconate or calcium chloride IV, correct acidosis, or hemodialyze

HYPOCALCEMIA *(calcium below 8.5 mEq/L)*
- Muscle tremors
- Tetany
- Paresthesias
- Labored, shallow respirations
- Biliary colic
- Bronchospasms
- Respiratory arrest
- Muscle cramps
- Tonic/clonic seizures
- Paralytic ileus
- Alterations in normal blood clotting
- Wheezing
- Laryngospasms

Treatment

- Monitor cardiopulmonary status
- Magnesium sulfate
- Calcium PO or slowly IV
- Vitamin D

HYPERCALCEMIA *(calcium above 10.5 mEq/L)*

- Drowsiness
- Headache
- Apathy
- Confusion
- Coma weakness
- Renal calculi, with associated flank pain or thigh pain
- Lethargy
- Depression
- Irritability
- Personality changes
- Flaccidity

Treatment

- IV Saline
- Monitor potassium and magnesium levels
- Mithramycin, etidronate disodium
- Diuretics
- Use IV phosphate with caution

HYPOMAGNESEMIA

- Anorexia
- Vomiting
- Delirium, confusion
- Digitalis-induced dysrhythmias
- Prolonged QT interval
- Coma
- Nausea
- Muscle tremors
- Convulsions
- Torsades de pointes
- ST depression

Treatment
- Magnesium sulfate 33 mEq IV over 5-10 min *(if renal function okay)*

HYPERCHLOREMIA
- Dysrhythmias
- Fatigue, leg cramps
- Irritability
- Respiratory distress
- Muscle weakness
- Drowsiness
- Shallow respirations
- Coma

Treatment
- Treat underlying cause

HYPOCHLOREMIA
- Decreased level of sensorium
- Tremors
- Muscle irritability
- Slow, shallow respirations

Treatment
- Chloride supplementation

HYPERPHOSPHATEMIA
- Muscle tremors
- Tetany
- Paresthesias
- Lengthened Q-T interval, lengthened S-T segment
- Wheezing
- Laryngospasms
- Dysrhythmias
- Muscle cramps
- Tonic/clonic seizures
- Paralytic ileus
- Alterations in normal blood clotting
- Bronchospasms
- Respiratory arrest
- Hypotension

- Biliary colic
- Positive Chvostek's and Trousseau's signs

Treatment
- Aluminum hydroxide gels
- Acetazolamide

- Normal T wave on EKG
- Labored shallow respirations

- Dialysis

HYPOPHOSPHATEMIA
- Malaise
- Anorexia
- Muscle wasting
- Hypoxia
- Vomiting
- Polyuria
- Shortened Q-T segment

- Confusion
- Muscle weakness
- Rhabdomyolysis
- Nausea
- Polydipsia
- Shortened Q-T interval
- Cardiac dysrhythmias

Treatment
- Phosphate PO or IV
- Treat cause

- No phosphate-binding gels

HYPERMAGNESEMIA
- Respiratory depression
- Apathy
- Areflexia
- Presence of peaked T wave and narrow QRS
- Abdominal cramping

- Lethargy
- Confusion
- Numbness to extremities
- Muscle flaccidity and paralysis
- Nausea

- Diarrhea
- Bradycardias
- Death ensues with levels of 6 mEq/L or more
- Oliguria
- Lethal dysrhythmias
- Muscle weakness
- Prolonged PR interval and QRS widening as condition worsens

Treatment
- Calcium chloride IV slowly

ENDOCRINE SYSTEM
GLANDS AND HORMONES SECRETED

Pituitary Glands

Anterior pituitary *(adenohypophysis)*
- Growth hormone (GH)
- Melanocyte-stimulating hormone (MSH)
- Follicle-stimulating hormone (FSH)
- Luteinizing hormone (LH)
- Interstitial cell-stimulating hormone (ISH)
- Prolactin (PR)
- Adrenocorticotropic hormone (ACTH)
- Thyroid-stimulating hormone (TSH)

Posterior pituitary *(neurohypophysis)*
- Antidiuretic hormone (ADH) (vasopressin)
- Oxytocin hormone

Hypothalamus
- Growth hormone-releasing hormone (GRH, GHRH)
- Growth hormone-inhibiting hormone (GIF, GHIH)
- Corticotropin-releasing hormone (CRH)
- Thyrotropin-releasing hormone (TRH)
- Prolactin-releasing hormone (PRH)
- Prolactin-inhibiting hormone (PIF,PIH)
- Follicle-stimulating hormone-releasing hormone (FRH)
- Luteinizing hormone-releasing hormone (LRH)

Thyroid Gland
- Thyroxin (T$_4$)
- Triiodothyronine (T$_3$)
- Thyrocalcitonin

Parathyroid Gland
- Parahormone (PTH)

Pancreas
- Insulin
- Glucagon

Adrenal Glands

Adrenal cortex [sugar, salt, sex]
- Androgens (sex)
- Glucocorticoids (sugar)
- Mineralocorticoids (salt)

Adrenal medulla
- Catecholamines (epinephrine and norepinephrine)

ENDOCRINE PROBLEMS

Thyroid Crisis (thyroid storm)
- Hypermetabolism from increased amounts of hormones
- Hyperthermia
- Diaphoresis
- Increased stroke volume

- Increased heart rate
- Increased cardiac output, with high output failure
- Decreased peripheral vascular resistance
- Atrial fibrillation, atrial or ventricular dysrhythmias
- Systolic murmur
- Widening pulse pressure
- Mild edema
- Tremors
- Bruit/thrill over thyroid
- Nausea/vomiting/diarrhea
- Confusion

Treatment:

- Administer oxygen
- Control temperature
- Monitor for dysrhythmias
- Plasmapheresis
- Medications: iodine (SSKI, Lugol's solution), glucocorticoids, propranolol, propylthiouracil, methimazole

Adrenal Crisis

- Low amounts to no cortical hormone present
- Sodium decreased
- Chloride decreased
- Potassium increased

- Urine sodium increased
- BUN increased
- Serum ACTH increased
- Serum cortisol decreased
- Serum calcium increased
- Urine cortisol decreased
- Weight loss
- Weakness and dehydration
- Hypotension
- Anorexia/nausea/vomiting
- Abdominal pain

Treatment:
- Administer IV fluids (saline) in large volumes
- Monitor I&O, cardiac monitor
- Medications: IV/IM cortisol, desoxycorticosterone, aldosterone

Diabetes Insipidus (DI)
- Deficiency in utilization or secretion of antidiuretic hormone
- Abrupt onset of polyuria (up to 24 L/day)
- Plasma osmolality increased
- Serum sodium increased
- Urine osmolality decreased
- Specific gravity decreased
- Plasma antidiuretic hormone decreased

- Continual thirst
- Weakness and dehydration
- Fever
- Confusion
- Hypotension
- Tachycardia
- Dehydration

Treatment:
- Administer IV/PO fluids (hypotonic initially)
- Monitor I&O Q hourly and replace output and specified amount IV)
- Weigh Q day
- Monitor VS and for dehydration
- Medications: vasopressin, desmopressin (DDAVP), lypressin, oral hypoglycemics
- Thiazide diuretics (if primary problem not reversible)

SYNDROME OF INAPPROPRIATE ANTIDIURETIC HORMONE (SIADH)
- Unexplained increases of vasopressin (ectopic production from oat cell CA)
- Hyponatremia
- Urine sodium increased
- Plasma osmolality decreased
- Specific gravity increased
- Weight gain without overt edema
- Weakness

- Lethargy
- Confusion
- Convulsions
- Coma

Treatment:
- Restrict fluids
- Monitor weight and I&O
- Monitor for bowel complications
- Monitor for electrolyte imbalances
- Medications: hypertonic saline, furosemide, lithium, demeclocycline, phenytoin sodium, urea

DIFFERENCES BETWEEN PRERENAL, RENAL AND POSTRENAL FAILURE

Prerenal	Renal	Postrenal
Urine output < 20 cc/hr	Variable	< 20 cc/hr
Bun/Creatinine > 10:1	> 20:1	> 20:1
Specific gravity > 1.020	Cortical: varies Medullary: 1.010	Varies
Urine protein minimal to none	Cortical: moderate to heavy Medullary: minimal to moderate	Moderate
Urine sodium < 20 mEq/L	> 40 mEq/L	> 20 but < 40 mEq/L
Urine osmolality > 450 mOsm/kg or > 100 mOsm more than plasma	< 350 mOsm/kg or = to plasma	< 400 mOsm/kg
Urine/Plasma osmolality > 1.5:1	< 1:1	< 1:1
Urine/serum creatinine > 40	< 20	< 20
Urine/plasma urea ratio >10:1	< 4:1	< 8:1
Urine sediment normal sediment	Cortical erythrocyte casts, leukocytes Medullary renal epithelial cells, tubular casts, rare erythrocyte	Few sediments

DIFFERENCES BETWEEN PRERENAL, RENAL AND POSTRENAL FAILURE

Prerenal	Renal	Postrenal
Causes		
Hypotension, Hypovolemia, Decreased cardiac output, Inadequate perfusion, Hemorrhage, Burns, Renal artery infarct, Aortic aneurysm	Acute tubular necrosis, Renal ischemia, trauma, Massive hemorrhage, Uremic syndrome, Nephrotoxins, Crush injuries, Septic shock, Cardiogenic shock, Glomerulonephritis, Good pasture's syndrome, Endocarditis, Malignant hypertension, Diseases of renal blood vessels, Systemic lupus erythematosus	Prostatic hypertrophy, Renal calculi, Abdominal tumors, Neurogenic bladder, Urethral obstructions, Obstructions at bladder neck or ureters, Bladder stone

Glomerular Filtration Rate (GFR)

$$GFR = \frac{\text{urine creatinine} \times \text{urine volume in cc/min}}{\text{plasma creatinine}}$$

Normal GFR = 125 cc/min

$$\text{Serum Osmolality} = (Na \times 2) + \frac{BUN}{3} + \frac{Glucose}{18}$$

$$\text{Plasma Osmolality} = 2(Na + K) + \frac{BUN}{3} + \frac{Glucose}{18}$$

NEUROLOGIC SYSTEM

TABLE OF CONTENTS

Glasgow Coma Scale 399
Initial Management of Head Injury Patients 400
Pupillary Size 400
Pediatric Coma Scale 401
Best Verbal Response 402
Neurologic Problems 403
Grading Systems of Deep Tendon Reflexes 406
Cranial Nerves 407
Autonomic Nervous System Reactions 408

GLASGOW COMA SCALE (GCS)

Eyes Open
- Spontaneously   4
- To verbal stimuli   3
- To pain   2
- Never   1

Best Verbal Response
- Oriented and converses   5
- Disoriented and converses   4
- Inappropriate words   3
- Incomprehensible sounds   2
- No response   1

Best Motor Response
- Obeys   6
- Localizes pain   5
- Flexion withdrawal   4
- Flexion (decorticate)   3
- Extension (decerebrate) 2
- No response   1

Glasgow coma scale scores may range from 3 to 15. For a score of 9 or less; the doctor should be notified. A score of 13 or less in a previously rated 15 patient, an unconscious patient, focal weakness, and/or unequal pupil size should be related to the doctor.

INITIAL MANAGEMENT OF HEAD INJURY PATIENTS

- Keep head in neutral position until cervical fracture is ruled out.
- Endotracheal intubation for all patients with GCS scores of 7 or less.
- Nasogastric drainage if appropriate (when patient vomits or has endotracheal intubation)
- Maintain PaO_2 of at least 90 mm Hg and pH of at least 7.4.
- Hyperventilation until $PaCO_2$ reaches 25 to 28 mm Hg.
- Administer glucocorticoids (at the discretion of the neurosurgeon).
- Administer dehydrating agents (at the discretion of the neurosurgeon).
- Stop bleeding from scalp and other external sites. (Shock is NOT due to head injury.)
- Treat hypotension with Ringer's lactate. DO NOT use 5% dextrose in water. Avoid overhydration. If patient is normotensive, administer maintenance fluids.

PUPILLARY SIZE

- Darken room prior to the examination of the pupils
- Pupil reaction time is normally brisk, examples of reaction time choices are: brisk, slow, or fixed (unresponsive)
- Pupils should react equally to light

PEDIATRIC COMA SCALE

Eyes Opening	Score	Over 1 Year	Less Than 1 year
	4	Spontaneously	Spontaneously
	3	To verbal command	To shout
	2	To pain	To pain
	1	No response	No response
Best Motor Response		**Over 1 Year**	**Less than one year**
	6	Obeys	
	5	Localizes pain	Localizes pain
	4	Flexion withdrawal	Flexion withdrawal
	3	Flexion—abnormal (decorticate)	Flexion —abnormal (decorticate)
	2	Extension (decerebrate)	Extension (decerebrate)
	1	No response	No response

Best Verbal Response		Over 5 Years	2-5 Years	0-23 Months
	5	Oriented, converses	Appropriate words and phrases	Smiles, coos, cries appropriately
	4	Disoriented, converses	Inappropriate words	Smiles, babbles recognizes family
	3	Inappropriate words	Cries and/or screams	Turns head to sound, recognizes family
	2	Incomprehensible sounds	Grunts	Grunts No response
	1	No response	No response	

Normal ICP is 4 to 15 mm Hg or 5 to 20 cm H_2O***
Important elevations of ICP should be reported to the physician if the pattern is significant for > 10 to 15 minutes duration cerebral perfusion pressure:

$$CPP = MAP - ICP$$

Normal 60-90 mm Hg

NEUROLOGIC PROBLEMS

Epidural Hematoma

An epidural hematoma is bleeding between the skull and the dura mater in the epidural space; possible causes include tears in the wall of the middle meningeal artery, or transverse or superior sagittal sinus and is often associated with linear skull fractures. Possibly caused by a blow to the head, this is the most serious complication of a head injury because the temporal lobe is forced down and inward which can cause uncal herniation and possibly death

Symptoms

Localized headache, restlessness, possible nausea/vomiting, ipsilateral pupil changes, contralateral motor paralysis, short period of unconsciousness, followed by a period of lucidness and alertness, may progress to coma.

Subdural Hematoma

A subdural hematoma is bleeding between the dura mater and the arachnoid into the subdural space, usually caused by venous bleeding; possible causes include a laceration of the brain with tear in the arachnoid that allows blood and CSF to collect into the subdural space, a ruptured saccular aneurysm or intracerebral hemorrhage; may occur spontaneously if the patient has dysfunctional coagulation.

Symptoms

Progressive change in level of consciousness, hemiparesis, ipsilateral pupil change, contralateral hemiparesis or hemiplegia, possible ipsilateral hemiparesis, extraocular eye movement paralysis, irritability, confusion, positive Babinski reflex and seizures

Subarachnoid Hematoma

A subarachnoid hematoma is bleeding in the subarachnoid space; possible causes include injury to a surface vessel in the subarachnoid space, congenital aneurysm, or arteriovenous malformation.

Symptoms

Sudden, violent headache, dizziness *(vertigo)*, tinnitus, facial pain, unilaterally dilated pupil, nuchal rigidity, hemiparesis, hemiplegia, nausea, vomiting, drowsiness, sweating, and chills.

Uncal (Tentorial) Herniation

A uncal herniation occurs when expanding lesions force the uncus of the temporal lobe over the medial edge of the tentorium; possible causes include a portion of the temporal lobe slipping into the posterior fossa related to a temporal lobe or a lateral extracerebral lesion; this exerts pressure on the third cranial nerve and eventually on the brain stem.

Symptoms

Ipsilateral loss of direct reaction to light, ipsilateral ptosis, ipsilateral losses of medial rectus muscle movement, contralateral loss of consensual reaction to light; pupil is usually small at first, then becomes progressively larger and fixed; motor paralysis affecting functionally-related groups of muscles, spasticity, hyperactive deep tendon reflexes in involved limbs, loss of cutaneous abdominal and cremasteric reflexes on paralyzed side, Babinski reflex on paralyzed side, atrophy and fasciculations of involved muscles, loss of doll's eye reflex; decerebrate rigidity, hyperthermia, and ataxic respirations.

Tonsillar (Medullary) Herniation
Downward displacement of the brain's posterior fossa; possible causes include cerebellar tonsils pressing through foramen magnum to the medullas possible causes include due to an expanding lesion of the hemispheres or a centrally-located extracerebral lesion; the brain stem distortion may lead to medullary collapse and death

Symptoms
Altered level of consciousness, nuchal rigidity, upper motor neuron involvement, frequent sighs and yawns that may lead to Cheyne-Stokes respiration patterns and hyperventilation , decorticate posturing, positive Babinski, bilateral pupil dilation, wide fluctuations in body temperature, flaccidity, respiration and circulatory collapse

GRADING SYSTEMS OF DEEP TENDON REFLEXES

GRADE	REFLEX RESPONSE
0	(0) absent
1	(+) sluggish or diminished
2	(++) active or normal
3	(+++) slightly hyperactive or increased response
4	(++++) brisk with intermittent or transient clonus
5	(+++++) very brisk with sustained clonus

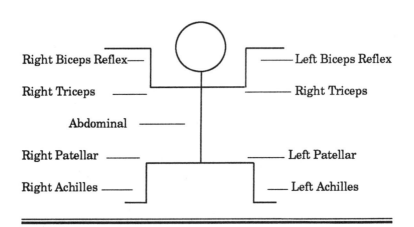

Right Biceps Reflex —
Right Triceps ———
Abdominal ———
Right Patellar ———
Right Achilles ———
— Left Biceps Reflex
— Right Triceps
— Left Patellar
— Left Achilles

Cranial Nerves

Number	Nerve	Symptoms of Defect
I	Olfactory	Unable to detect a specific odor
II	Optic	Defect in visual fluid
III	Oculomotor	Droopy eyelid, lack of consensual pupil response
IV	Trochlear	Nystagmus, wandering eye(s)
V	Trigeminal	Unable to clench teeth, absence of blinking, decreased sensation to forehead, eyes, nose, sinuses, teeth, jaw, tongue or ear
VI	Abducens	Diplopia on lateral gaze
VII	Facial	Asymmetrical facial movement, loss of taste on anterior ⅔ of tongue
VIII	Acoustic	Loss of hearing and balance, difficulty with coordination of head and eye movements
IX	Glossopharyngeal	Loss of taste impaired gag reflex, nasal speech; impaired reflex control of respiration, pulse, and blood pressure
X	Vagus	Difficulty swallowing, loss of voice, orthostatic hypotension, slow heart rate
XI	Spinal Accessory	Weakness of trapezius and sternocleidomastoid muscles
XII	Hypoglossal	Twitching of tongue, dysphagia

A mnemonic useful, in remembering these cranial nerves is: On Old Olympus Towering Top, a Finn And German Viewed Some Hops.

AUTONOMIC NERVOUS SYSTEM REACTIONS

Body Part	Sympathetic Reaction	Parasympathetic Reaction
Bladder	Acts with parasympathetic system in voiding	Contracts bladder muscle, relaxes sphincter
Blood pressure	Increases	Decreases or no reaction
Bronchioles	Dilates	Constricts
Coronary vessels	Dilates	No significant action
Gastrointestinal muscle	Inhibits peristalsis, stimulates sphincter, relaxes smooth muscles	Stimulates peristalsis, inhibits sphincter contracts smooth muscles
Heart rate	Increases	Decreases
Penis	Causes ejaculation	Causes erection
Pupils	Dilate	Constricts
Responses of body systems	Widespread, systemic	Localized
Salivary gland	Thick, viscous secretions	Watery secretions
Skeletal muscle vessels	Constricts	Dilates

PEDIATRICS

TABLE OF CONTENTS

Physiologically Unstable Infants 411
Cardiopulmonary Assessment 412
Signs and Symptoms of Deterioration 413
Dysrhythmias in Children 415
Approximate Children's Dosages 417
Basic Life Support in Children 418
Information for Pediatric Emergency
Medications 424
Maintenance Calories 427
Calculation of Drug Dosages 427
Determining Drug Adminstration Rates with
Variable Drug Concentrations 428
Modification of Maintenance Fluid
Requirements Based on Condition 430
Congenital Heart Defects 433

PHYSIOLOGICALLY UNSTABLE INFANTS

Recognizing a physiologically unstable infant or child may be difficult but can be done by direct physical examination alone. Lab tests may be helpful in confirming the presence of deterioration or the severity of the condition, but should not be relied on for the diagnosis of instability. A rapid cardiopulmonary assessment can be done in 30 seconds or less and should be done to assess pulmonary and cardiovascular integrity with any of the following conditions:

- Respiratory rate > 60
- Heart rate > 140 (under 5 years) > 120 (over 5 years)
- Respiratory distress, dyspnea
- Trauma
- Hemorrhage
- Burns
- Cyanosis
- Failure to recognize parents
- Diminished level of consciousness
- Seizures
- Fever with petechiae
- Admission to an ICU

CARDIOPULMONARY ASSESSMENT

A rapid cardiopulmonary assessment consists of:

AIRWAY PATENCY

Breathing Rate

Air entry
   Chest expansion
   Chest symmetry
   Breath sounds
   Stridor
   Wheezing

Mechanics
   Sternal retractions
Nasal flaring
   Grunting
   Cyanosis

CIRCULATION

Heart Rate

Blood pressure
Peripheral pulses
   Present/absent
   Volume amplitude

Skin perfusion
   Capillary refill time
   Temperature
   Color
   Mottling
CNS perfusion
   Recognition of parents
   Response to pain
   Muscle tone
   Presence of seizures
   Pupil size/equality

SIGNS AND SYMPTOMS OF DETERIORATION:

(Note: *Atropine may mask hypoxia-induced bradycardia*)

- Decreasing activity level
- Drooling
- Sternal retractions
- Noisy respirations
- Irritability
- Increased work of breathing
- Orthopnea
- Fatigue with normal activity
- $pO_2 < 100$ on 100% O_2
- Bradycardia (late sign)
- Cold, mottled extremities
- Dysrhythmias
- Child does not "look right" or "normal" to parents
- Cyanosis of oral mucosa or periphery
- Poor feeding
- Nasal flaring
- Restlessness
- Air hunger
- Respiratory pattern changes
- $S_aO_2 < 90$
- $pCO_2 > 50$
- Tachycardia (early sign)
- Prolonged capillary refill time
- Hypotension (late sign)

Procedures that put a child at risk for deterioration:

- **Suctioning**—causes hypoxia and decreases the mean airway pressure leading to atelectasis or vagal responses

- **Chest physiotherapy**—mobilizes secretions that may not be handled well creating respiratory distress
- **Lumbar puncture**—may compress the airwayS or cause a vagal response, or herniation may occur (if cerebral edema is present)

Procedure that produces vagal stimulation
- Sedation (may assist or worsen condition)
- When oxygen support is removed
- Feedings
- Over stimulation and stress
- Transport

Ways of Compensating for Respiratory Failure:
- Increasing minute volume
- Increasing effort
- Expiratory grunting
- Pursed lip breathing
- Increasing V/Q matching
- Acid-base regulation
- Hyperventilation
- Increasing oxygen consumption
- Increasing hemoglobin
- Increasing cardiac output *

(*Children cannot increase their stroke volume, they can increase only rate)

DYSRHYTHMIAS IN CHILDREN

	ST	SVT	A Flutter	VT
Patient History	Sepsis, fever, hypovolemia	Usually normal	Majority have an abnormal heart	Majority have an abnormal heart
Atrial Rate	Almost always less than 230/min	Majority greater than 230/min 260-300=infant	Atrial 250-500 vent. conduction 1:1 to 4:1	Usually rate less than 250=child 200-500=infants
Variation in Ventilation Rate	May speed up or slow down over several seconds	Usually very regular after first 10-20 beats	May have variable degree or block	Slight variation over several beats

DYSRHYTHMIAS IN CHILDREN

	ST	SVT	A Flutter	VT
P Wave Axis	Same as sinus, almost always P waves visible	Most have visible P waves, but these waves do not look like sinus P waves	Flutter waves	May have AV dissociation, retrograde or absent P waves
QRS Complexes	Almost always the same as with the slower sinus rhythm	After first several beats, almost always the same as sinus rhythm	Usually same as sinus, but may have different beats	Different from sinus, not necessarily wide and bizarre complexes

APPROXIMATE CHILDREN'S DOSAGES

This is a rough estimate of approximates based on fractions of an adult dose and does not take individual size or specific medicine into account. For accurate dosing, each medicine should be reviewed.

AGE	FRACTION OF ADULT DOSE
1 month	$1/20$
3 months	$1/15$
6 months	$1/10$
9 months	$1/9$
1 year	$1/7$
2 years	$1/6$
3 years	$1/5$
4 years	$1/4$
5-6 years	$1/3$
7-8 years	$1/2$
10-12 years	$2/3$
13-15 years	$3/4$

BASIC LIFE SUPPORT IN CHILDREN

Airway—essential to successful pediatric resuscitation

Breathing

    Infants—20 breaths per minute (< 1 yr)

    Children—15-20 breaths per minute (1-8 yrs)

    Children—15 breaths per minute (> 8 yr)

Circulation

    Check pulses:
- Infants
  - Brachial/femoral
- Children
  - Carotid

Compression

    Infants: 2-3 fingers, one finger-breadth below the nipple line on the lower third of the sternum at rate of 100/minute

    Child: heel of one hand on the lower third of the sternum at the rate of 100/minute

Compression

    Ventilation ratio 5:1 for all children and infants

AIRWAY/BREATHING

The airway of a child differs from that of an adult in many ways—the upper airway is smaller and more flexible, the tongue is relatively larger, the glottic opening is higher, the smallest diameter of the airway is at the cricoid cartilage rather than the vocal cords, the lower airways are smaller and more easily obstructed, and a child's metabolic rate is usally twice that of an adult.

OXYGEN DELIVERY

The nasal cannula is unsuitable for children in an emergency since FIO_2 cannot be controlled and since humidification cannot be provided. Nasal catheter use is discouraged since it has no advantage over the nasal cannula and it may cause hemorrhage from trauma or gastric distention. The oxygen tent cannot provide a satisfactory FIO_2 over 30% and the mist makes it difficult, to assess the child without opening the tent and lowering the FIO_2. Oxygen masks are not tolerated by infants or young children, and a face tent does not allow reliable FIO_2, concentrations in excess of 40%. The oxygen hood is the best type of delivery system since it allows visualization of most of the body and has a quicker recovery rate for the FIO_2

AIRWAYS

An *oropharyngeal airway* can be useful in maintaining patency in an unconscious child or infant, if other measures to open the airway fail to provide and unobstructed airway. The oropharyngeal airway can stimulate retching and vomiting in a conscious patient and an improper sized airway may actually cause obstruction. In children and infants, the oral airway **should not** be inserted and rotated the way it is in the adult—instead a tongue blade should be used to prevent damage to place airway and the oral cavity. A *nasopharyngeal airway* is better tolerated in conscious patients. The outside diameter should not be so large as to cause blanching of the outer sides of the nostril, or so small that nasal airways may become obstructed by mucus, blood, vomitus or the soft tissues of the pharynx.

Endotracheal airways are required when prolonged ventilation is needed, or when adequate ventilation cannot be achieved with a mask-bag-valve device. Cuffed ET tubes are indicated only in children over 8 years old. Children under 8 years of age utilize their narrowing at the cricoid ring as a functional cuff for an ET tube. A straight blade for the laryngoscope is used in infants and children up to 8 yrs because it provides greater displacement of the tongue into the floor of the mouth and better visualization of the glottis. Proper positioning of the tube should be confirmed by observation of symmetrical chest expansion, auscultation of equal bilateral breath sounds, and absence of breath sounds over the stomach, observation of condensation in the ETT during expiration, and positively by chest x-ray.

ABNORMAL RHYTHMS

In infants and children, arrhythmias should be treated as an emergency only if they compromise cardiac output or they have the potential for degenerating into a rhythm that compromises cardiac output. When rapid rates produce cardiovascular instability, they should be treated by synchronized cardioversion. In non-emergency situations, these rapid rhythms can be managed with other methods. The slow rhythms associated with acute cardiopulmonary emergencies usually result from atrioventricular block or suppression of normal impulse generation caused by a combination of acidosis and hypoxemia. Usually, cardiac arrest in children is due to respiratory dysfunction or arrest. Initial therapy consist of proper ventilation and oxygenation, with medication such as atropine if needed.

SVT

This rapid regular rhythm is better tolerated in older children but can cause cardiovascular collapse with clinical shock in infants. The heart rate is usually around 240/min in infants but can be as high as 300/min and is usually due to a reentry mechanism. In severely ill infants, it may be difficult to distinguish sinus tachycardia from SVT. In ST, usually heart rate is less than 200/min

VT

Heart rate may vary from almost normal to more than 400/min. Slow rates may be tolerated, but the more rapid rates compromise cardiac output and may degenerate into VF. The majority of children with VT have structural heart disease or a prolonged Q-T interval.

BRADYCARDIA

Every slow rhythm associated with poor cardiac output is first treated by ensuring good ventilation and oxygenation. Medications such as atropine and epinephrine can then be used.

VF

Ventricular fibrillation is extremely rare in infants and uncommon in children unless there is underlying congenital cardiac disease. Defibrillation should be carried out quickly once diagnosis of VF is assured, with 1 watt/sec per pound or 2 watt/sec per kilogram of body weight. If initial defibrillation is unsuccessful, the amount may be doubled to 4 watt/sec/kg and defibrillated twice. If the pediatric patient has been in VF longer than 2 minutes, basic life support with CPR should be performed for 2 minutes before defibrillation is attempted.

VENTILATORY SUPPORT

With volume ventilators, children have a higher airway resistance, smaller airway diameter, and a smaller tidal volume. Some problems with volume ventilators concerning the pediatric patient include poor coordination between the ventilator and the child's effort, premature delivery systems, and inadequate I:E ratio that results in alveolar hypoventilation. The pO_2 should be at least 70 to 80 for a child. I:E ratio should be 1:1 or 1:2, PEEP 3 to 5 cm H_2O, and rate and FIO_2 dependent on the pathology of the child. Tidal volume is usually 5 to 7 cc/lb.

Neonatal ventilators have an IMV mode in which the infant receives a set FIO_2, as well as an end-expiratory pressure between mandatory breaths. This causes the infant to use the diaphragm and assists with weaning off the ventilator.

Pressure-limited ventilators allow the peak inspiratory pressure (PIP), inspiratory time and flow rate to be set. The problem with this is that the tidal volume is determined by the PIP **and** the patient's lung compliance so that the tidal volume is variable. Being able to control the PIP lessens the chance of barotrauma but may result in hypoventilation.

Volume-limited ventilators allow the tidal volume and inspiratory time to be set which enables a constant volume to be delivered. The PIP is variable and can be measured by the pressure gauge. Being able to control the volume lessens the chance of alveolar rupture, but areas of decreased compliance and lung collapse are under-ventilated, and in infants with large areas of atelectasis, this may cause intrapulmonary shunting and hypoxemia.

The choice between these types of ventilators is based on physician and hospital preference.

NORMAL VALUES	HR	RESP	BP
Infant	140-160	40	60
Preschooler	120-140	30	SBP = 80 + 2 (age in years)
School age	100-120	20	DBP = 2/3 of SBP

INFORMATION FOR PEDIATRIC EMERGENCY MEDICATIONS

MEDICATION	STANDARD DOSE
Adenosine	0.1-0.2 mg/kg IV; Maximum single dose: 12 mg
Atropine	0.02 mg/kg IV or may be given via ET tube; Minimum single dose: 0.1 mg; Maximum dose: 1.0 mg
Bretylium	5 mg/kg IV; may increase to 10 mg/kg
Bicarbonate (sodium)	1 mEq/kg/dose or base deficit × kg × 0.3; Maximum dose: 8 mEq/kg/24 hrs
Calcium Chloride (10%)	20 mg/kg/dose IV slowly; Maximum infusion rate: 100 mg/min
Calcium Gluconate (10%)	100 mg/kg/dose IV; Maximum infusion rate: 100 mg/min
for defibrillation:	2 W/s/kg; Reduce dose if patient is digitalized

INFORMATION FOR PEDIATRIC EMERGENCY MEDICATIONS

MEDICATION	STANDARD DOSE
Epinephrine *for bradycardias:* *for code:*	0.01 mg/kg (of 1:10,000 solution) IV or intraosseous 0.1 mg/kg (of 1:1000 solution) ET tube 0.01 mg/kg (of 1:10,000 solution) IV or intraosseous 0.1 mg/kg (of 1:1000 solution) ET tube Subsequent dose 0.1-0.2 mg/kg (1:1000 solution) IV, intraosseous, or ET tube
Epinephrine infusion	0.1 µg/kg/ min
Furosemide (lasix)	1 mg/kg/dose IV; Maximum dose: 5-10 mg
Glucose (50% Or 25%)	1 cc/kg dose of $D_{50}W$ or 2 cc/kg/dose of $D_{25}W$
Lidocaine (xylocaine)	Bolus: 1 mg/kg/dose IV; Drip: 20-50 µg/kg/min
Mannitol (25% Osmitrol)	0.15-0.5 g/kg/dose IV (150-500 mg/kg/dose)
Morphine	0.1 mg/kg/dose IV or subq
Naloxone (narcan)	0.01 mg/kg/dose/IV (10 mg/kg/dose)
Pancuronium (pavulon)	Loading: 0.05 mg/kg IV; Maintenance: 0.1 mg/kg/hr
Potassium Chloride	0.5-1 mEq/kg/dose IV; diluted in solution Administer over 2-4 hours

INFORMATION FOR PEDIATRIC EMERGENCY MEDICATIONS

MEDICATION	STANDARD DOSE
Additional Medications	
Medication	Concentration (µg/cc)
Dobutamine (Inotrex)	150 mg/250 cc = 600 µg/cc
Dopamine (Intropin)	150 mg/250 cc = 600 µg/cc
Epinephrine (Adrenalin)	1 mg/100 cc = 10 µg/cc
Isoproterenol (Isuprel)	0.5 mg/100 cc = 5 µg/cc
Lidocaine (Xylocaine)	120 mg/100 cc = 1,200 µg/cc
Nitroglycerine	150 mg/250 cc = 600 µg/cc
Sodium nitroprusside (Nipride)	10 mg/100 cc = µg/cc

May wish to double concentration and adjust rate for larger children on some medications

Endotracheal (ET) Tube Size:
$$\frac{\text{Age (in years)}}{4} + 4 = \text{size in mm}$$

Circulating Blood Volume (CBV) 80 cc/kg in infants
70 cc/kg in children

MAINTENANCE CALORIES
(TOTAL DAILY REQUIREMENT)
- Neonate: 125 calories/kg/day
- Infant: 100 calories/kg/day
- Toddler: 90 calories/kg/day
- Preschooler: 85 calories/kg/day
- School-age child: 75 calories/kg/day
- Adolescent: 60 calories/day

CALCULATION OF DRUG DOSAGES
Using the Rules of 6's:
- For dopamine (and other drugs requiring dosages of approximately 1-20 µg/kg/minute:
- 6.0 × body weight (in kg) = _____mg added to diluent to total 100 cc (concentration = _____mg/100 cc)

Then the cc/hr provided of this solution will equal the µg/kg/minute of the solution given (i.e., if this solution is run at 5 cc/hr, the patient will receive 5 µg/kg/minute of the drug)

- For epinephrine, isoproterenol, sodium nitroprusside (and other drugs requiring dosages of less than 1-20 µg/kg/minute:
- 0.6 × body weight (in kg) =____ mg added to diluent to total 100 cc (concentration = mg/100 cc)

Then, the cc/hr provided of this solution will equal the tenths of a µg/kg/minute of the solution given (i.e., if this solution, is run at 7 cc/hr, patient will receive 0.7 µg/kg/minute of the drug).

DETERMINING DRUG ADMINISTRATION RATES WITH VARIABLE DRUG CONCENTRATIONS

- To determine dosage of a known concentration of drug that child is receiving:
  - If concentration is X mg/Y cc, divide X by Y to yield a concentration of drug in mg/cc. Then multiply that number by 1000, to provide the number of µg of the drug per cc.
  - Multiply the µg/cc times the rate of infusion (cc/hr) to determine the micrograms per hour the child is receiving.
  - Divide the µg/hour by 60 to yield the µg/minute.
  - Divide the µg/minute by the child's weight in kilograms to yield the µg/kg/minute the child is receiving.

- To determine how many cc/hour of a known concentration will provide a given dose (x µg//kg minute) of a vasoactive drug
  - To determine µg/kg/min:

$$\mu g/kg/min = \frac{mg/cc \times 1000\,\mu g/mg \times IV\ rate\ (cc/hr)}{60\ min/hr \times P+ W+ (kg)}$$

  - To determine µg/min:

$$\mu g/min = \frac{mg/cc \times 1000\,\mu g/mg \times IV\ rate\ (cc/hr)}{60\ min/hr}$$

  - To deliver desired µg/min:

$$cc/hr = \frac{\mu g/min\ desired \times 60\ min/hr}{\mu g/cc\ concentration\ of\ available\ solution}$$

— To determine mg/min:
$$mg/min = \frac{mg/cc \times IV\ rate\ (cc/hr)}{60\ min}$$
— To deliver desired mg/min:

$$cc/hr = \frac{mg/min\ desired \times 60\ min/hr}{mg/cc\ (concentration\ of\ available\ solution)}$$

— Multiply desired dose (× μg/kg/minute) by child's weight to obtain the μg/minute of the drug the child should receive
— Multiply the μg/minute of the drug by 60 and this yields the μg/hour the child should receive
— Determine the concentration of the drug at hand (divide mg present by volume of solution), then convert this concentration to μg/cc
— Divide the total μg/hour the child should receive by the number of μg present in each cc of fluid; this will yield the rate (in cc/hr) of administration of the drug.
— Rate of infusion is (To determine rate to provide desired μg/kg/min) desired

$$cc/hr = \frac{kg \times dose\ (\mu g/kg/min) \times 60\ min/hr}{\mu g/ml\ (or\ available\ concentration\ solution)}$$

MODIFICATION OF MAINTENANCE FLUID REQUIREMENTS BASED ON CONDITION

If the child has pulmonary, cardiovascular, or renal disease, or if increased intracranial pressure is present, fluid administration rates should be reduced.

If the child is dehydrated, has fever, or other causes of increased insensible water losses, fluid requirements will be increased. Overbed warmers or bililights increase evaporative fluid losses. Fever increases insensible water losses approximately 10 cc/kg/degree centigrade elevation in temperature above 37 degrees for a 24-hour period.

Mild Dehydration

5% weight loss or up to 50 cc/kg. Symptoms include sunken eyes, dry mucous membranes, poor skin turgor, depressed fontanelles, tachycardia with normal blood pressure and respiratory rate. Child looks ill, and may be irritable or restless.

Treatment

Replace fluid deficit (up to 50 cc/kg or 1/2 maintenance fluid requirements) while providing maintenance fluid requirements.

Moderate Dehydration

5-10% weight loss or up to 100 cc/kg. Symptoms include: tachycardia, tachypnea, cool and clammy skin, dry mucous membranes, eyes sunken, depressed fontanelles, decreased peripheral pulses, decreased urine output. Child may be irritable or lethargic.

Treatment

Replace fluid deficit (up to 100 cc/kg or 1 × maintenance fluid requirement) in addition to provision of maintenance fluid requirements.

Severe Dehydration

More than 10% weight loss or up to 150 cc/kg. Symptoms include: obtundation, hypotension, metabolic acidosis, and signs of shock.

Treatment

Provide resuscitation of intravascular volume while maintaining electrolyte balance; then replace fluid deficit (up to 150 cc/kg or 1 ½ × maintenance fluid requirements) while providing maintenance fluid requirements.

Hypotonic Dehydration

Fluid loss is primarily from the intravascular compartment symptoms include poor systemic perfusion than is more severe with smaller fluid deficits.

Treatment

Replace half of the calculated deficit, in addition to maintenance fluid requirements, during the first 8 hours of therapy and the remaining half of the fluid deficit, in addition to the normal maintenance fluid requirements, during the next 16 hours *(Deficit replacement should be given only after resuscitation of intravascular volume and restoration of effective perfusion is accomplished.)*

Hypertonic Dehydration

Fluid loss is primarily from the extravascular compartment, so intravascular volume is maintained at the expense of fluid shift from the cells and the interstitial space. Symptoms include: milder hypovolemic symptoms despite relatively large volume deficits.

Treatment

Replacement of fluid deficit is accomplished gradually over 48 hours, and care should be taken to prevent rapid falls in serum sodium concentration during rehydration.

CONGENITAL HEART DEFECTS

Ventricular Septal Defect (VSD)

An opening in the ventricular septum that allows blood to shunt from the left ventricle to the right ventricle; most common congenital defect

Signs and symptoms
- Fatigue
- Pale
- Thin, frail looking
- Dyspneic
- Tachypneic
- Difficulty with feeding
- Poor growth pattern
- Harsh systolic murmur best heard at the 3rd and 4th intercostal spaces to the left of the sternum
- Palpable thrill over the upper left sternal border
- Increased right ventricular and pulmonary artery pressures
- PMI displaced laterally
- Left sided heart failure increased PVR
- Shunt can reverse with time to right to left shunt

On Chest X-ray
- Left atrial and left ventricular enlargement
- Dilated pulmonary artery

On EKG
- Left atrial hypertrophy
- Left ventricular hypertrophy
- Right ventricular hypertrophy

Treatment
- Defect may close spontaneously after 6 months of age
- Asymptomatic patients do not require surgery
- Corrective surgery performed after age 1 year or if shunt is greater than 2:1

Atrial Septal Defect (ASD)

An opening between the left and right atria that allows blood to shunt from left to right between chambers; caused by delayed or incomplete closure of the foramen ovale or atrial septal wall

Signs and symptoms
- Dyspnea with exertion (especially in infants)
- Orthopnea
- Fatigue
- Frail, delicate appearance
- Increased number of respiratory infections
- Left precordial bulge
- Soft midsystolic murmur best heard at 2nd or 3rd intercostal space
- Possible diastolic murmur
- Fixed split of S2
- Shunt can reverse with pulmonary hypertension to a right to left shunt
- Pulmonary artery may rupture
- Can result in pulmonary embolism

On Chest X-ray
- Right atrial and right ventricular enlargement
- Right atrial and right ventricular volume overload

On EKG
- Atrial fibrillation and/or flutter
- Atrial dysrhythmias
- Right bundle branch blocks
- Right axis deviation (secundum, sinus venosus)
- Left axis deviation (primum)
- Right atrial hypertrophy
- Right ventricular hypertrophy

Treatment
- Defect may close spontaneously within 1 year of birth
- Corrective surgery performed after 1 year of age or for shunts greater than 1.5:1

Patent Ductus Arteriosus (PDA)

Patent ductus arteriosus is an opening between the aorta and the pulmonary artery bifurcation that fails to close after birth and allows shunting from the left to right (from the pulmonary artery to the aorta); this normally closes within 72 hours after birth; can be associated with coarctation of the aorta, and cause aneurysm of the ductus

Signs and symptoms
- Cyanosis to lower parts of the body
- Pink color to the upper parts of the body
- Clubbing of toes
- Feeds poorly
- Fatigue
- Increased number of respiratory infections
- Systolic thrill palpable at the 2nd intercostal space

- Bounding pulses (with large defects)
- Loud continuous murmur at the left upper sternal border (machinery—like murmur)
- Widened pulse pressure
- Pulmonary congestion

On Chest X- ray
- Left atrial and left ventricular enlargement
- Enlargement of the aorta
- Left sided heart overload

On EKG
- Left atrial and left ventricular hypertrophy

Treatment
- Medical management with a prostaglandins inhibitor, domethacin
- Digoxin (controversial)
- Control congestive heart failure
- Restriction of fluids and salt
- Diuretics
- PEEP
- Corrective surgery performed

Tetralogy of Fallot

A combination of 4 defects, those being a ventricular septal defect, overriding aorta, pulmonary stenosis and right ventricular hypertrophy

Signs and symptoms
- Cyanosis
- Finger and toe clubbing
- Dyspnea
- Syncope

- Limpness convulsions (occasionally)
- Child assumes a squatting position (flaccid or lateral knee—chest in infants)
- Respiratory distress during feeding
- Growth is retarded
- Loud systolic murmur best heard over the left sternal border
- Possible cardiac thrill palpable at the left sternal border

[can be associated with iron deficiency anemia, polycythemia, abscesses, coagulation disorders, or cerebral infarcts]

Treatment
- Corrective surgery if cyanosis occurs before 3 months of age
- Corrective surgery after age 1 year, usually at 4-5 years of age

Coarctation of the Aorta (COA)

A narrowing of the aorta usually distal to the left subclavian artery; associated with bicuspid aortic valves

Signs and symptoms
- Dizziness, fainting, headache
- Epistaxis
- Cold feet
- Leg cramps
- Increased BP and bounding pulses proximal to the defect
- Hypotension and weak or absent pulses distal to the defect (cardinal sign of COA)
- Upper body more developed than lower body

- Palpable arteries over the precordium and between the ribs
- Soft high frequency murmur at sternal border.
- Pulmonary hypertension
- Systolic ejection click at the base and apex
- Systolic or continuous murmur between the scapulae
- Aneurysm proximal to the defect
- Hypertrophy of the left ventricle
- S_3
- Left ventricular pressures increased
- Increased afterload

On chest X-ray
- Left ventricular enlargement
- Rib notching on 4th through the 8th ribs

On EKG
- Left ventricular and/or right ventricular hypertrophy

Treatment
- Corrective surgery between 3 to 5 years of age if no associated elevation in upper extremity pressures > 140 mm Hg.

WEIGHTS AND MEASURES

TABLE OF CONTENTS

Temperature Equivalents 441
Frequently Used Equivalents in the Metric System . 443
Standard Basal Calories 445
Abdominal Anatomic Sites 446
Clotting Factors and Their Synonyms 447
Symptoms and Possible Poisons 448
Miscellaneous Signs and Symptoms 461
Blood Type Compatibility 470
What to Chart 471

TEMPERATURE EQUIVALENTS

Centigrade	Fahrenheit
34.0	93.2
34.2	93.6
34.4	93.9
34.6	94.3
34.8	94.6
35.0	95.0
35.2	95.4
35.4	95.7
35.6	96.1
35.8	96.4
36.0	96.8
36.2	97.1
36.4	97.5
36.6	97.8
36.8	98.2
37.0	98.6
37.2	98.9
37.4	99.3
37.6	99.6
37.8	100.0
38.0	100.4
38.2	100.7
38.4	101.1
38.6	101.4
38.8	101.8

39.0	102.2
39.2	102.5
39.4	102.9
39.6	103.2
39.8	103.6
40.0	104.0
40.2	104.3
40.4	104.7
40.6	105.1
40.8	105.4
41.0	105.8
41.2	106.1
41.4	106.5
41.6	106.8
41.8	107.2
42.0	107.6
42.2	108.0
42.4	108.3
42.6	108.7
42.8	109.0
43.0	109.4

To convert degrees Centigrade to degrees Fahrenheit:
($9/5 \times$ temperature) + 32

To convert degrees Fahrenheit to degrees Centigrade:
(temperature - 32) $\times 5/9$

FREQUENTLY USED EQUIVALENTS IN THE METRIC SYSTEM

1 gram (g, gm,)	= 0.001 kilogram(kg)
	= 0.01 hectogram(hg
	= 0.1 decagram(dag)
	= 10 decigrams (dg)
	= 100 centigrams (cgg)
	= 1,000 milligrams (mg)
1 liter (L, l)	= 0.001 kiloliter (kl)
	= 0.01 hectoliter (hl)
	= 0.1 dekaliter (dal)
	= 10 deciliters (dl)
	= 100 centiliters (cl)
	= 1,000 milliliters (ml)
	= 1,000 cubic centimeters (cc)
1,000 mg	= 15 grains
600 mg	= 10 grains
500 mg	= 7.5 grains
300 mg	= 5 grains
100 mg	= 3 grains
60 mg or 65 mg	= 1.5 grains
45 mg	= ¾ grain
30 mg	= ½ grain

15 mg	=	¼ grains
1 mg	=	¹⁄₆₀ grain
0.6 mg	=	¹⁄₁₀₀ grain
0.5 mg	=	¹⁄₁₂₀ grain
0.4 mg	=	¹⁄₁₅₀ grain
0.3 mg	=	¹⁄₂₀₀ grain
1 teaspoonful	= 1 fluidram	= 4 or 5 ml
1 tablespoonful	= ½ fluid ounce	= 15 ml
2 tablespoonful	= 1 fluid ounce	= 30 ml
1 cup	= 8 fluid ounces	= 240 ml
1 pint	= 16 fluid ounces	= 480 ml
1 quart	= 32 fluid ounces	= 960 ml
1 gallon	= 128 fluid ounces	= 3,840 ml

20 grains	= 1 scruple
3 scruples	= 1 dram
8 drams	= 1 ounce
16 ounces	= 1 pound

60 minims	= 1 fluidram
8 fluidram	= 1 fluid ounce
16 fluid ounces	= 1 pint
2 pints	= 1 quart
4 quarts	= 1 gallon

STANDARD BASAL CALORIES

AGE	WT. (Kg)	Kcal/Kg/24 hrs. caloric expenditure
Newborn	2.5-4	50
1 wk-6 mo	3-8	65-70
6 mo-12 mo	8-12	50-60
1 yr-2 yr	10-15	45-50
2 yr-5 yr	15-20	45
5 yr-10 yr	20-35	40-45
10 yr-16 yr	35-60	25-40
Adult	70	15-20

Add 12% of the standard basal calories for each degree of temperature rectally above 37.8 °Centigrade

ABDOMINAL ANATOMIC SITES

Right Hypochondriac	Epigastric	Left Hypochondriac
Right lobe of liver Gallbladder Part of duodenum Hepatic flexure of colon Part of right kidney Suprarenal gland	Pyloric end of stomach Duodenum Pancreas Aorta Portion of liver	Stomach Spleen Tail of pancreas Splenic flexure of colon Upper pole of left kidney
Right Lumbar	**Umbilical**	**Left Lumbar**
Ascending colon Lower half of right kidney Part of duodenum Jejunum	Omentum Mesentery Transverse colon Lower parts of jejunum, duodenum, and ileum	Descending colon Lower half of left Kidney Parts of jejunum and ileum
Right Iliac	**Hypogastric**	**Left Iliac**
Cecum Lower end of ileum Right ureter Right spermatic cord Right ovary	Ileum Bladder Uterus	Sigmoid colon Left ureter Left spermatic cord Left ovary

CLOTTING FACTORS AND THEIR SYNONYMS

Factor	Synonym
I	Fibrinogen
Ia	Fibrin
II	Prothrombin
IIa	Thrombin
III	Thromboplastin
IV	Calcium
V	Acglobulin (labile factor, proaccelerin)
VII	Proconvertin (Autoprothrombin I)
VIIa	Convertin
VIII	Amtihemophiliac globulin (AHG)(Antihemophillic Factor) IX
	Christmas factor (Autoprothrombin II) Plasma thromboplastin component (PTC)
IXa	Activated PTC
X	Stuart-Power factor (Autoprothrombin III)
XI	Plasma thromboplastin antecedent (PTA)
XII	Hageman factor
XIIa	Activated Hageman factor
XIII	Fibrin-stabilizing factor

SYMPTOMS AND POSSIBLE POISONS

When the poison agent is unknown, clinical observation of the patient may be valuable for ascertaining the possible toxic substance ingested. This is by no means an all inclusive list.

Eyes

Signs/Symptom	Poisons
Pupillary dilatation	Belladonna alkaloids, atropine, glutethimide, meperidine, sympathomimetics, parasympatholytics, antihistamines, cocaine, camphor, benzene, botulism toxin, cyanide, carbon monoxide, LSD, mescaline, thallium, alcohols, tricyclics
Pupillary constriction	Opiates, sympatholytics, parasympathomimetics, barbiturates, cholinesterase inhibitors, chloral hydrate, phenothiazines, ethanol, organophosphate insecticides, phencyclidine (PCP)

Eyes

Signs/Symptoms	Poisons
Nystagmus	Phenytoin, phencyclidine, (PCP), barbiturates, sedatives, tricyclic antidepressants
Ptosis	Botulism toxin, phenytoin
Strabismus	Botulism toxin, thallium

Face and Scalp

Signs/Symptoms	Poisons
Alopecia	Arsenic, radioactive agents, cancer chemotherapy, vitamin A, lead, boric acid, thallium
Facial twitching	Lead, mercury

Skin and Mucous Membranes

Signs/Symptoms	Poisons
Sweating	Cholinergics, organophosphate insecticides, nicotine, phencyclidine (PCP)
Hypothermia	Ethchlorvynal, barbiturates
Hot, dry skin	Atropine, belladonna alkaloids, botulism toxin, sympathomimetics, amphetamines
Flushing	Sympathomimetics, anticholinergics, boric acid, carbon monoxide, alcohol, snake bites, atropine, antihistamines, phenothiazines, disulfuram
Salivation	Caustics, arsenic, mercury, bismuth, cholinergics, organophosphate insecticides, muscarine-containing mushrooms, salicylates, nicotine, fluoride, phencyclidine (PCP)

Skin and Mucous Membranes

Signs/Symptoms	Poisons
Dry mouth	Atropine, belladonna alkaloids, botulismtoxin, antihistamines, sympathomimetics, narcotics, anticholinergic
Burns	Corrosives, thallium, boric acid, phenols
Stomatitis	Cancer chemotherapy
Pink (cherry)	Carbon monoxide, cyanides, boric acid
Yellow	From hepatic injury (chlorinated compounds, heavy metals, mushrooms, and several drugs), from hemolytic anemias, aniline, fava beans, quinacrine, vitamin A

Skin and Mucous Membranes

Signs/Symptoms	Poisons
Cyanotic, (without respiratory depression or shock)	Nitrobenzene, chlorates, carbon dioxide, ethylene glycol, iron, nitrites, nitrates, ergot, and numerous other drugs and chemicals, methemoglobinemias
Red orange	Rifampin

Nervous System

Signs/Symptoms	Poisons
Obtundation, coma	Opiates, all hypnotics, sedatives and general anesthetics, barbiturates, chloral hydrate, belladona, paraldehyde, chloroform, flurazepam ethers, bromides, alcohols, lead, cyanide, carbon monoxide, carbon dioxide, nicotine, benzene, atropine, scopolamine, some cholinesterase inhibitors, insulin, aniline

Nervous System

Signs/Symptoms	Poisons
Obtundation, coma (continued)	derivatives, mushrooms, salicylates, propoxyphene anticonvulsants, phencyclidine (PCP)
Delirium, agitation	Atropine, belladonna alkaloids, cocaine, alcohol, caffeine, lead, marijuana, arsenic, amphetamines, antihistamines, phenothiazines, phecyclidine camphor, LSD, (PCP), benzene, barbiturates, DDT, aniline dyes, theophylline, digitalis, tricyclic antidepressants, phenytoin
Convulsions	Strychnine, camphor, cocaine, atropine, belladonna alkaloids, organophosphate insecticides, amphetamines, nicotine, lead, phenols mushrooms, caffeine, theophylline, cyanides, tricyclic anti-depressants, salicylates, narcotics, barbiturate withdrawal, boric acid,

Nervous System

Signs/Symptoms	Poisons
	Mercury, phenothiazines, antihistamines, arsenic, DDT, hydrocarbons, fluoride, digitalis, thallium, alcohols, phencyclidine (PCP), propoxyphene, phenytoin
Headache	Organophosphate insecticides, carbon monoxide, benzene, anilines, lead, caffeine, cocaine
Muscle spasms	Atropine, strychnine, lead, spider and scorpion bites, phenothiazines, camphor, fluorides, phencyclidine (PCP)
Paresthesias weakness, paralysis	Carbon monoxide, botulism toxin, alcohols, curare, DDT, nicotine, cyanide, mercury, lead, arsenics, thallium, organophosphates, fluoride

GI Tract

Signs/Symptoms	Poisons
Nausea, vomiting, diarrhea, abdominal pain	Arsenic, iron, corrosives, lead, spider bites, boric acid, organophosphates, phosphorus, nicotine, fluorides, thallium, methanol, mushrooms, digitalis, opiates, DDT, botulism toxin, cocaine, salicylates, theophylline, snake venom, food poisoning, mercury, naphthalene, disulfiram
Dysphagia	Caustics, fluoride, iron, arsenic, salicylates, theophylline, warfarin, phosphorus, phenytoin

Ear

Signs/Symptoms	Poisons
Tinnitus	Salicylates, quinine, quinidine, aminoglycosides, camphor, nicotine, methanol, diuretics, lithium (mild)

Renal

Signs/Symptoms	Poisons
Proteinuria	Arsenic, mercury, phosphorus
Hematuria and/or hemoglobinuria	Arsenic, mercury, naphthalene, other hemolytic oxidizers, cyclophosphamides

Hematologic

Signs/Symptoms	Poisons
Anemia	Lead, naphthalene, other hemolytic agents, snake venom
Hemorrhage	Warfarin, thallium, snake venom
Methemoglobinemia	Nitrates, nitrites, anilines
Rhabdomyolysis	Barbiturates

Respiratory

Signs/Symptoms	Poisons
Respiratory depression/failure	Opiates, fluorides, cyanides, barbiturates, alcohols, snake venom, carbon monoxide, benzodiazepines, phenothiazines, organophosphate, ethclorvynol
Tachypnea/hyperpnea	Atropine, belladonna alkaloids, cocaine, amphetamines, strychnine, salicylates, camphor, hydrocarbons, snake venoms, cyanides, carbon monoxide, talc, caustics
Dyspnea	Cyanides, carbon monoxide, carbon dioxide, snake venoms, benzene, acetone

Cardiovascular

Signs/Symptoms	Poisons
Bradycardia	Digitalis, mushrooms, quinine, quinidine, lead, barbiturates, opiates, organophosphates, beta- blockers
Tachycardia	Amphetamines, atropine, belldonna alkaloids, cocaine, sympathomimetics, caffeine, theophylline, phenothiazines, antihistamines
Hypertension	Amphetamines, sympathomimetics, lead, nicotine, cortisone, cocaine
Hypotension	Chloral hydrate, glutethimide, phenothiazines, iron, sympathomimetics, tricyclic antidepressants, phenytoin, ethchlorvynol, alcohols, lithium

Cardiovascular

Signs/Symptoms	Poisons
Cardiovascular Collapse	Leads, acids, alkalis, opiates, phenols, endotoxins, food poisoning, iron, amphetamines, mushrooms, disulfiram, barbiturates
Dysrhythmias	Digitalis, tricyclic antidepressants, theophylline, narcotics, amphetamines, phenothiazines, solvents, antihistamines

Breath Odors

Signs/Symptoms	Poisons
Alcoholic	Phenols, chloral hydrate, alcohol
Sweet	Chloroform, acetone, ether
Bitter almond	Cyanides
Pears	Chloral hydrate

Breath Odors

Signs/Symptoms	Poisons
Garlic	Phosphorus, arsenic, organophosphate insecticides
Violets	Turpentine
Pine	Pine oil

General

Signs/Symptoms	Poisons
Fever	Atropine, salicylates, food poisoning, antihistamines, phenothiazines, camphor, alcohols, theophylline, quinine, belladonna alkaloids

MISCELLANEOUS SIGNS AND SYMPTOMS

Allis' sign

- Relaxation of the fascia between the iliac crest and the greater trochanter when pressing firmly with a finger over the area with the finger sinking deeply; possible indication of a fracture of the neck of the femur. Also, unequal leg lengths seen in congenital hip dislocation.

Amoss' sign

- A maneuver to avoid pain with flexion of the spine demonstrated by supporting oneself by placing the hands far behind the person after rising from a lying to a sitting position.

Argyll Robertson pupil

- A small, irregular pupil that constricts normally in accommodation but poorly, if at all, in response to light: possible indication of chronic syphillitic meningitis or other forms of syphillis

Balances' sign

- A mass or area of dullness found by palpation or percussion of the left upper quadrant of the abdomen: possible indication of hematoma following a splenic rupture

Ballet's sign

- Paralysis of the external ocular muscles causing the loss of control of voluntary eye movement but normal reflexive movement and pupillary light reflexes: are present possible indication for thyrotoxicosis

Barre's pyramidal sign
- The inability to hold the lower legs still with the knees flexed; possible indication of pyramidal tract disease

Beau's lines
- Transverse linear depressions on the fingernails; possible indication for malnutrition, nail trauma, coronary artery occlusion, or toxic reactions

Beevor's sign
- Upward movement of the umbilicus upon contraction of the abdominal muscles; possible indication of paralysis of the lower recti abdominous muscles usually associated with T 10 lesions.

Bitot's spots
- White or gray spots appearing on the conjunctiva at the lateral margin of the cornea; positive indication of vitamin A deficiency

Blepharoclonus
- Excessive blinking of the eyes; positive indication of disorders of the basal ganglia and cerebellum

Blumberg's sign
- abdominal pain caused by abrupt relese of steady pressure (rebound tenderness) over suspected abdominal lesion; possible indication of peritonitis or peritoneal inflammation

Bozzolo's sign
- Pulsation of the arteries in the nasal mucous membranes; possible indication of thoracic aortic aneurysm

Braunwald sign
- A weak pulse immediately after a premature ventricular contraction; possible indication of idiopathic hypertrophic subaortic stenosis (IHSS)

Broadbent's inverted sign
- Pulsation on the left posterolateral chest wall during ventricular systole; possible indication of gross dilation of left atrium

Broadbent's sign
- Visible retraction of the left posterior chest wall near the 11th and 12th ribs, occurring during systole; possible indication of adhesive pericarditis

Chaddock's sign
- Dorsiflexion of the great toe when the foot is stroked around the lateral malleolus and along the dorsum laterally; positive indication of pyramidal tract lesions

Coopernail sign
- Ecchymoses on the perineal, scrotal, or labial areas; possible indication of pelvic fracture

Corrigan's pulse
- A jerky pulse with a strong surge then an abrupt collapse; possible indication of aortic insufficiency, severe anemia, coarctation of the aorta, systemic arteriosclerosis, or patent ductus arteriosus

Cullen's sign
- A bluish hemorrhagic discoloration around the umbilicus and occasionally around an abdominal scar; possible indication of massive intraperitoneal hemorrhage after trauma or rupture, or in acute hemorrhagic pancreatitis

Darier's sign
- Wheals and itching of the skin after rubbing macular lesions; positive indication of release of histamine when mast cells are irritated

Delbet's sign
- No pulses palpable in the distal portion of a limb, in conjunction with normal color and temperature; possible indication of aneurysmal occlusion of a main artery

Dorendorf's sign
- Fullness at the supraclavicular groove; possible indication of aortic arch aneurysm

Duchenne's sign
- The inward movement of the epigastrium during inspiration; possible indication of diaphragmatic paralysis or pericardial effusion

Duroziez's sign
- A double murmur heard over the femoral artery or other large peripheral artery; possible indication of aortic insufficiency

Erb's sign
- Dullness on percussion over the manubriumof the sternum; possible indication of tetany

Ewart's sign
- Bronchial breathing auscultated with dullness upon percussion below the angle of the left scapula; possible indication of pericardial effusion

Glabella reflex
- Persistent blinking in reponse to repetitive light tapping on the forehead between the eyebrows; possible indication of Parkinson's disease, presenile dementia or frontal lobe tumors

Grey Turner's sign
- A bruise like discoloration of the skin of the flanks; possible indication of acute pancreatitis

Hamman's sign
- A loud crushing, crunching sound synchronous with the heart beat; possible indication of mediastinal emphysema that occurs with pneumothorax or rupture of the trachea or bronchi

Hemorrhage (subungual)
- Hemorrhagic lines or bleeding under the nail; possible indication of subacute bacterial endocarditis or trichinosis

Hill's sign
- A femoral systolic pulse pressure 60 to 100 mmHg higher in the right leg than in the right arm: possible indication of severe aortic insufficiency

Homan's sign
- Deep calf pain with forced dorsiflexion of the foot; possible indication of thrombophlebitis

Hoover's sign

- The inward movement of one or both costal margins with inspiration; possible indication of emphysema with respiratory distress or intrathoracic disorders. Also, a test for hysterical paralysis. Examiner asks person to raise unaffected leg while placing hand under affected leg, pressure from affected leg is felt against examiners hand as unaffected leg is raised.

Janeway's spots (lesions)

- Slightly raised, irregular, non-tender erythematous lesions on the palms and soles; possible indication of infective endocarditis

Kashida's sign

- Increased sensitivity to and muscle spasms after the application of heat or cold, possible indication of tetany

Kehr's sign

- Referred left shoulder pain when the patient is supine; positive indication of peritoneal hemorrhage

Kernig's sign:

- Reflex contraction and pain in the hamstring muscles when attempting to extend the leg after flexing the thigh toward the body; symptom of meningitis

Kleist's sign

- Flexion of the fingers when passively raised; possible indication of frontal lobe and thalamic lesions

Kussmaul's sign

- Distention of the jugular veins on inspiration; possible indication of constrictive pericarditis or mediastinal tumor, also can refer to a paradoxical pulse that indicates absorption of toxins

Leichtenstern's sign

- Pain with gentle tapping of the bones of an extremity; possible indication of cerebrospinal meningitis

Lhermitte's sign

- Sensations of brief, sudden, electric-like shocks that spread down the back and into the extremities when the head is flexed forward; possible indication of multiple scierosis, spinal cord degeneration or cervical spinal cord injury

Macewan's sign

- A cracking pot-type sound heard after percussion with a single finger over the anterior fontanelle; possible indication of hydrocephalus or cerebral abscess

Murphy's sign

- When gentle pressure is applied to the gallbladder area, pain occurs during deep inspiration; possible indication of acute cholecystitis or hepatitis

Nicoladoni's sign

- Bradycardia results from finger pressure on an artery proximal to an AV fistula

Olocardiac reflex

- Bradycardia response to vagal stimulation by applying pressure to the eyeball or carotid sinus, possible diagnosis of angina or relief of angina pain

Orbicularis sign

- The inability to close one eye at a time (wink) ; possible indication of hemiplegia

Pastia's sign

- Petechiae that appear along the skin folds; possible indication of streptococcus toxin reactions

Perez's sign

- Crackles auscultated over the lungs when a patient raises and lowers his arms; possible indication of aortic aneurysm or fibrous mediastintis

Perez's reflex

- Mass reflex present at birth which consists of extension of the head and spine, flexion of the knees to the chest, a cry, and emptying of the bladder; absence of this reflex during first 3 months of life indicates serious neurological impairment

Piotrowski's sign

- Excessive dorsiflexion and supination of the foot with tapping of the anterior tibial muscle: possible indication of a central nervous system disorder

Pitres's sign

- Anterior deviation of the sternum; possible indication of pleural effusion

Potain's sign

- Dullness with percussion over the aortic arch; possible indication of aortic dilatation

Prevost's sign

- Conjugate deviation of the head and eyes (usually with the gaze toward the affected hemisphere); possible indication of hemiplegia

Quincke's pulse

- Alternate blanching and flushing of the nail bed; possible indication of aortic insufficiency

Quinquaud's sign

- Trembling of the fingers; possible indication of alcoholism

Rotch's sign

- Dullness on percussion over the right lung at the fifth intercostal space; possible indication in pericardial effusion

Roth's spots

- Round or oval white spots seen in the retina; possible indication of subacute bacterial endocarditis

Rumpel-Leeds' sign

- Petechiae distal to a tourniquet placed on the upper arm; possible indication of scarlet fever or thrombocytopenia

Signorelli's sign

- Extreme tenderness upon palpation of the area anterior to the mastoid, possible indication of meningitis

Vein sign

- A palpable, bluish cordlike swelling along the line formed in the axilla by the junction of the thoracic and the superficial epigastric veins, possible indication of tuberculosis or obstruction of the superior vena cava

BLOOD TYPE COMPATIBILITY

Blood Type	Compatible RBCs	Compatible Plasma
O	O	O, A, B, AB
A	A, O	A, AB
B	B, O	B, AB
AB	AB, A, B, O	AB
Positive Rh	+ or -	+ or -
Negative Rh	-	+ or -

WHAT TO CHART

Neurologic—level of consciousness, orientation, speech, behavior, pupil size, pupil equality, pupil reaction, blink, corneal, gag, and cough reflexes, cranial nerve-function, motor strength, gait, posture, vision and hearing, headache, dizziness, vertigo

Skin—texture, temperature, turgor, presence of lacerations, contusions, abrasions, open wounds, scars, pressure areas, color, rashes, ecchymoses, petechiae, growths, lesions

Cardiovascular—heart rate and rhythm, blood pressure, heart sounds and lung sounds, apical and peripheral pulses, activity tolerance, presence of Homan's sign, jugular vein distention, edema, rubs, bruits, murmurs, thrills, hums, gallops, acrocyanosis

Respiratory—breathing pattern and rate, shape of chest, symmetry of chest expansion, normal and adventitious breath sounds, exertion response work of breathing, cough, sputum characteristics, presence of pain, dyspnea, rubs, airways, tracheostomy, mechanical ventilation, chest tubes

Gastrointestinal—condition of teeth, gums, mucous membranes, abdominal pulsations and bruits, abdominal contour and symmetry, presence of scars, visible blood vessels, appetite, bowel habits, bowel sounds, stool, special diets, nutritional status, presence of abdominal distention, nausea, vomiting, pain

Genitourinary—breast shape and symmetry, genital inflammation, ulceration, discharge, breast tenderness or lumps, voiding patterns, urine color, consistency, odor, specific gravity, presence of flank pain, nocturia, discharge, incontinence, hematuria, urgency difficulty initiating or maintaining urinary stream

Musculoskeletal—range of motion, muscle strength presence of deformities, amputations, arthritis, spasms, cramping, tingling, atrophy, hypertrophy, paralysis, flaccidity

Other—presence and location of intravenous lines, IV fluids and other continuing medications, PA lines, catheters, drains, tubes, and characterisics of drainage from theses, IABP, arterial lines, method of oxygenation, treatments, wound care, appropriate waveforms from hemodynamic lines, pacemakers, including permanent, temporary, and external ones, airways, oximeter readings restraint devices, complaints from patient, care provided, instructions and teaching given, ability to retain and comprehend instructive process, return demonstrations, and follow up on previously noted findings.

APPENDIX: GLOSSARY OF ABBREVIATIONS

GLOSSARY OF ABBREVIATIONS

ABGs	Arterial blood gases
AC	Assist control, before meals
ACLS	Advanced cardiac life support
AED	Automatic external defibrillator
AF, Afib	Atrial fibrillation
Agap	Anion gap
AIVR	Accelerated idio-ventricular rhythm
AMI	Acute myocardial infarction
ANT	Anterior
ARDS	Adult respiratory distress syndrome
Art	Arterial
ASHD	Arteriosclerotic heart disease
AV	Arterio-venous, atrial-ventricular
BPM	Beats per minute
BSA	Body surface area
BUN	Blood urea nitrogen
CABG	Coronary artery bypass grant
CAD	Coronary artery disease
CHB	Complete heart block
CHF	Congestive heart failure
CHI	Closed head injury
CI	Cardiac index
CMV	Controlled mechanical ventilation

CO	Cardiac output, carbon monoxide
CO_2	Carbon dioxide
COP	Colloid osmotic pressure
COPD	Chronic obstructive pulmonary disease
CPAP	Continuous positive airway pressure
CPR	Cardiopulmonary resuscitation
CPP	Coronary perfusion pressure, cerebral perfusion pressure
CPT	Chest physiotherapy
CSF	Cerebrospinal fluid
CT	Computerized tomography, chest tube
CVD	Cardiovascular disease
CVP	Central venous pressure
Cx	Circumflex artery
CXR	Chest X-ray
DBP	Diastolic blood pressure
DIC	Disseminated intravascular coagulation
Dig	Digoxin
DJD	Degenerative joint disease
DI	Diabetes insipidus
DKA	Diabetic ketoacidosis
DM	Diabetes mellitus
DTR	Deep tendon reflexes
Dx	Diagnosis
ECG, EKG	Electrocardiogram

EEg	Electroencephalogram
EF	Ejection fraction
EMD	Electromechanical dissociation
EOA	Esophageal obturator airway
EDP	End-diastolic pressure
EDV	End-diastolic volume
ESRD	End-stage renal disease
ET, ETT	Endotracheal tube
ETOH	Ethyl alcohol
Ext	External
FIO_2	Fraction of inspired oxygen
FSP	Fibrin split products
Fx	Fracture
GCS	Glasgow coma scale
GSW	Gun shot wound
HA	Headache
Hct	Hematocrit
HD	Hemodialysis
Hep lock	Heparin lock
HFJV	High frequency jet ventilation
Hg	Mercury
Hgb	Hemoglobin
HHNC	Hyperglycemic hyperosmolar non-ketotic coma
HOB	Head of bed

HIV	Human immunodeficiency virus
HHN	Hand held nebulizer
HR	Heart rate
Hr, hrs	Hour, hours
HTN	Hypertension
IAB	Intra-aortic balloon
IABP	Intra-aortic balloon pump
ICP	Intracranial pressure
ICU	Intensive car unit
IDDM	Insulin-dependent diabetes mellitus
IHSS	Idiopathic hypertrophic subaortic stenosis
IM	Intramuscular
IMV	Intermittent mandatory ventilation
Inf	Infusion
Int	Internal
IPPB	Intermittent positive pressure breathing
IV	Intravenous
IVCD	Intra-ventricular conduction delay
IVP	Intravenous push, intravenous pyelogram
IVPB	Intravenous piggyback
JVD	Jugular vein distention
K, K^+	Potassium
KUB	Kidney, ureter, bladder

KVO	Keep vein open
LAD	Left anterior descending (artery), left axis deviation
LA	Left atrial, left atrium
LAHB	Left anterior hemiblock
Lat	Lateral
LBBB	Left bundle branch block
LCA	Left coronary artery
LE	Lupus erythematosus
LICS	Left intercostal space
LLL	Left lower lobe, left lower lung
LLQ	Left lower quadrant
LOC	Level of consciousness, laxative of choice
LPHB	Left posterior hemiblock
LSB	Left sternal border
LUL	Left upper lobe, left upper-lung
LUQ	Left upper quadrant
LVEDP	Left ventricular end diastolic pressure
LVEDV	Left ventricular end diastolic volume
LVH	Left ventricular hypertrophy
LVSW	Left ventricular stroke work
LVSWI	Left ventricular stroke work index
Lytes	Electrolytes
MABP, MAP	Mean arterial blood pressure, mean arterial pressure

MAT	Multifocal atrial tachycardia
MI	Myocardial infarction
MRI	Magnetic resonance imaging
MRSA	Methicillin resistant staphylococcus auresus
MSOF, MOF	Multi-system organ failure
Na	Sodium
NaCl	Sodium chloride
NC,N/C	Nasal cannula
NS	Normal saline
NIDDM	Non-insulin dependent diabetes mellitus
NG	Nasogastric
NKA	No known allergies
NPH	Neutral Protein Hagedorn (Insulin)
NPO	Nothing by mouth
NSAID	Non-steroidal anti-inflammatory drugs
NTG	Nitroglycerin
O_2	Oxygen
SaO_2	Oxygen saturation
OBS	Organic brain syndrome
OD	Right eye
OS	Left eye
OU	Both eyes
PA	Pulmonary artery
PAD	Pulmonary artery diastolic

PAM, PA	Pulmonary artery mean
PAP	Pulmonary artery pressures
PAS	Pulmonary artery systolic
PAWP	Pulmonary artery wedge pressure
PACs	Premature atrial contractions
PaO$_2$	Partial pressure of arterial oxygen
PAT	Paroxysmal atrial tachycardia
PCN	Penicillin
PD	Peritoneal dialysis
PEA	Pulseless electrical activity
PO$_2$	Partial pressure of oxygen
PaCO$_2$	Partial pressure of arterial carbon dioxide
PCO$_2$	Partial pressure of carbon dioxide
PCWP	Pulmonary capillary wedge pressure
PE	Pulmonary embolus
PEARL	Pupils equal and reactive to light
PERRLA	Pupils equal, round and reactive to light and accommodation
PEEP	Positive end expiratory pressure
pH	Hydrogen ion concentration
PIP	Peak inspiratory pressure
PJCs	Premature junctional contractions
PB	Phenobarbital
Plt	Platelets

Post	Posterior
PSV	Pressure support ventilation
PSVT	Paroxysmal supra-ventricular tachycardia
PT	Prothrombin time, pro time
PTT	Partial thromboplastin time
PVCs	Premature ventricular contractions
PVD	Peripheral vascular disease
PvO$_2$	Venous oxygen saturation
PVR	Pulmonary vascular resistance, peripheral vascular resistance
PVRI	Pulmonary vascular resistance index, peripheral vascular resistance index
RA	Right atrium, rheumatoid arthritis
RAD	Right axis deviation
RBBB	Right bundle branch block
RCA	Right coronary artery
Resp	Respirations, respiratory
RICS	Right intercostal space
RLL	Right lower lobe, right lower lung
RLQ	Right lower quadrant
RML	Right middle lobe, right middle lung
RSB	Right sternal border
RT	Respiratory therapy
RUL	Right upper lobe, right upper lung
RV	Right ventricle, right ventricular

Appendix: Glossary of Abbreviations

RVH	Right ventricular hypertrophy
RVSW	Right ventricular stroke work
RVSWI	Right ventricular stroke work index
SaO$_2$	Arterial oxygen saturation
SA	Sino-atrial
SB	Sinus bradycardia
SBP	Systolic blood pressure
SIADH	Syndrome of inappropriate antidiuretic hormone
SR	Sinus rhythm
ST	Sinus tachycardia
SG, Sp.gr.	Specific gravity
SL, Sl	Sublingual
SOB	Shortness of breath
SP	Suprapubic, status post
SQ	subcutaneous
SSS	Sick sinus syndrome
SV	Stroke volume
SVI	Stoke volume index
SvO$_2$	Mixed venous oxygen saturation
SVR	Systemic vascular resistance
SVRI	Systemic vascular resistance index
SVT	Supraventricular tachycardia
SW	Stroke work
SWI	Stroke work index

SX,Sx	Symptom
TEA	Endarterectomy
TIA	Transient ischemic attack
TPR	Temperature, pulse, respiration; total peripheral resistance
TPN	Total parenteral nutrition
VEA	Ventricular ectopic activity
VT	Tidal volume
VF	Ventricular fibrillation
VT	Ventricular tachycardia
WNL	Within normal limits
WPW	Wolff-Parkinson-White syndrome

WORKS CITED

Abels, Linda F. *Mosby's Manual of Critical Care*, St Louis: C.V. Mosby, 1979.

Alspach, JoAnn G., editor *Core Curriculum for Critical Care Nursing*, 4th edition, W.B Saunders, Philadelphia, 1991.

Berkow, Robert, editor. *The Merck Manual of Diagnosis and Therapy*, 14th edition, Merck, Sharp, and Dohme Research Lab, Rahway, NJ, 1982.

Braunwald, E., et al, editor. *Harrison's Principles of Internal Medicine*, 11th edition, New York, McGraw-Hill Book Co., 1987.

Burns, Carol, Crawford, Mac. "A Method for Rapidly Calculating Intravenous Drip Rate," *Focus on Critical Care*, August 1988

Carmichael, R.M. *Notes from inservices on ABGs, Ventilators, EKGs, Medical conditions, 1989, 1990, 1991.*

Datascope Corporation. *Intra-Aortic Balloon Pump Manual*, Montvale, NJ, 1990.

Deepake, V., Babcock, R., and Magilligan, D. "A Simplified Concept of Complete Physiological Monitoring of the Critically Ill Patient", *Heart and Lung 10 (1) 75-82*

Directory of Tests and Services. Damon Clinical Laboratory, Needham Heights, 1993.

Dublin, Dale. *Rapid Interpretation of EKGs*, Cover Publishing Co.

Medtronic, Inc. *Pacing Glossary*, Medtronic, 1988.

Meltzer, Lawrence, et al. *Intensive Coronary Care*, 4th edition, Robert Brady Co., 1983.

Milne, Barbara. "Guide to Common Antihypertensive Drugs", *Nurses Review*, Volume 2, Vascular Problems, 8-89, Springhouse Book Co., 1986.

Minssen, Beth. Notes from Panhandle Education for Nurses's Seminars, 1990.

Nurse's Reference Library, Nursing 81-82 Books, Intermed Communications, Inc. *Assessment, Definitions, Drugs, Signs and Symptoms, Diagnostics, and Diseases.*

Shilling, Esther. "External Pacemaker: What the Nurse Needs to Know", *Medtronic News* (June 1982).

Shoemaker, William, et al. *Textbook of Critical Care*, Philadelphia: W.B. Saunders Co., 1984.

Skidmore-Roth, Linda. *Diagnostic and Laboratory Cards*, 2nd edition, El Paso: Skidmore-Roth Publishing, 1993.

Stapleton, John F. *Essentials of Clinical Cardiology* Philadelphia. F.A. Davis Co., 1983.

Urban, N. "Integrating Hemodynamic Parameters with Clinical Decision Making", *Critical Care Nurse*, 6 (2), 48-61.

Urban, N. "Cardiac Output/Cardiac Index Algorithm", Proceedings from NTI 1988, 135.

Woods, Susan L., editor. *Cardiovascular Critical Care Nursing,* New York: Churchill-Livingstone Co., 1983.

Wincek, Hazinski, and Moloney-Harmon. Notes taken from pre-NTI Pediatric Workshop, NTI 1988.

The ICU Quick Reference

INDEX

A

A wave, 263, 265
A/G ratio, 3
Abdominal anatomic sites, 445
Abducens nerve, 407
Ablation, 317
Acebutolol, 59
Acetaminophen, 3, 52
Acid phosphatase, 3
Acoustic nerve, 407
Acquired immune deficiency syndrome (AIDS), 369
Acromegaly, 41, 43-44
Activated coagulation time (ACT), 3
Activity threshold, 317
Acute pericarditis, 312
Acyclovir sodium, 61
Addison's disease, 41, 182, 374, 376
Addisonian crisis, 378
Adenocard, 63
Adenosine, 63, 424
Adrenal crisis, 390
Adrenal glands, 389
    Adrenal cortex, 389
    Adrenal medulla, 389
Adrenalin Chloride, 117
Adrenalin Chloride Solution, 117
Adrenergic, 139, 173
Adrenergic direct-acting beta-1 agonist, 113
Adult respiratory distress syndrome (ARDS), 267, 351, 357, 354, 369
    ARDS physiology, 369

Afterload, 255, 335
Agonist, 115
Airway, 418
Airway patency breathing, 412
Alanine aminotransferase (ALT), 4
Alatone, 197
Alazine, 134
Albumin, 42
Albumin, serum, 4
Aldactone, 197
Aldomet, 151
Algorithms, 233
Alkaline phosphatase, 4
Alkalinizer, 195
Allis' sign, 461
Alpha-1 antitrypsin, 4
Alpha-2 Macroglobulin, 5
Alteplase, 65
Alveolar ventilation, 347
Alveoli, 348
Amino acid screen, urine, 5
Ammonia, plasma, 5
Amodopa, 151
Amoss' sign, 461
Ampere, 317
Amphotericin B, 51, 67
Ampicillin, 52
Amrinone lactate, 70
Amylase, serum, 5
Amylase, urine, 5
Ancef, 86
Anesthetic, 146
Angina, 59, 189
Anion gap, 33
Anion gap (AGAP), 33
    High, 34

Low, 33
Normal, 34
Anti-DNase B Titer, 6
Anti-infective, 137
Anti-smooth muscle antibody (ASMA), 6
Anti-strep screen, 6
Anti-strep titer, 6
Anti-Thrombin III Assay, 6
Antianginal, 166
Antiarrhythmic, 59
Antibacterial, 119
Antibacterial macrolide, 100
Antibiotics, 84, 86, 88, 92, 94, 96, 132, 142, 175, 201
Anticonvulsants, 149, 177
Antidysrhythmics, 63, 108, 126, 162, 184, 187, 192, 203
Antidysrhythmics (Class B), 158
Antifungals, 128
Antifungal antibiotic, 67
Antihypertensive, 82, 106, 144, 151, 155, 160, 166, 171, 183, 199
Antinuclear antibody titer (ANA), 6
Antithrombotics, 65
Anturane, 48
Aortic aneurysm, 334
Apogen, 132
Apresoline, 134
Argyll Robertson pupil, 461
Arterial line, 331
Arterial oxygen content, 352
Ascites, 130
Aspartate aminotransferase (AST), 6
Aspergillosis, 67
Aspirin, 48, 52
Assist control (AC), 355
Assisted aortic end-diastolic pressure, 335

Assisted systole, 335
Asystole, 75, 240
Atenolol, 72
Atrial extrasystoles, 59
Atrial fibrillation, 390
Atrial septal defect (ASD), 434
Atrial systole, 336
Atromid, 48
Atropine, 74, 239-240, 424
Augmented unipolar leads, 295
Autonomic nervous system, 408
 Parasympathetic, 256
 Sympathetic, 256
AV block
 First degree, 309
 Second degree, Type I, 309
 Second degree, type II, 309
 Third degree, 309
AV conduction deficits, 309
Axis determination, 304

B

Bacteremia, 88
Bacteria, 39
Balances' sign, 461
Ballet's sign, 461
Barre's pyramidal sign, 462
Basophils, 35
Beau's lines, 462
Beck's triad, 268
Beevor's sign, 462
Bence Jones Protein, 7
Betaloc, 155
Bicarbonate, 7, 43
Bicarbonate (sodium), 424
Bilirubin, direct, serum, 7
Bilirubin, fecal, 7
Bilirubin, indirect, serum, 7
Bilirubin, micro, 7

Bilirubin, total, 7
Bilirubin, urine, 8
Bitot's spots, 462
Blastomycosis, 67
Bleeding time, 8
Blepharoclunus, 462
Blocadren, 199
Blood pressure
   Diastolic, 270
   Systolic, 266, 268, 270
Blood type compatibility, 470
Blood urea nitrogen (BUN), 8, 43
Blumberg's sign, 462
Body surface area (BSA), 257, 259
Bone metastases, 40-41, 43
Bradycardia, 242-243, 294, 378, 382, 458
Bradydysrhythmias, 75
Bradypnea, 351
Braunwald sign, 463
Breath sounds, 365-366
   Bronchial, 365
   Normal, 365
   Vesicular, 365
Breathing, 418
Bretylate, 77
Bretylium, 237, 424
Bretylium tosylate, 77
Bretylol, 77
Brevibloc, 122
Broadbent's inverted sign, 463
Bronchitis, 368
Bronchophony, 366
Bumetanide, 79
Bundle branch block, 294
   Left, 305
   Right, 305
Butazolidine, 48
Buzzolo's sign, 463

C

c wave, 263, 265, 314
C-Reactive protein quantitative, 15
Calan, 207
Calan SR, 207
Calcium, 40
   Daily approximate requirements, 376
Calcium chloride, 81, 424
Calcium gluconate, 424
Calcium, serum, 8
Calcium, urine, 8
Calcium, urine screen, 8
Calcium-channel blocker, 81, 207
Capoten, 82
Captopril, 82
Carbamazepine level, 9
Carbon dioxide, 9
Carcinoma, 45
Cardiac arrest, 195
Cardiac catheterization
   Complications of, 341
Cardiac cycle, 314
Cardiac glycoside, 108
Cardiac index (CI), 258
Cardiac inotropic agent, 70
Cardiac output (CO), 258
Cardiac tamponade, 268, 340
Cardiogenic shock, 333
Cardioquin, 192
Cardiovascular, 458, 471
Cascara sagrada, 50
Catapres, 106
Cefamandole naftate, 84
Cefazolin, 86
Cefazolin sodium, 86
Cefotaxime sodium, 88
Cefoxitin sodium, 90

Ceftazidime, 92
Ceftriaxone sodium, 94
Cefuroxime sodium, 96
Cena-K, 180
Centigrade, 441
Central venous pressure (CVP), 258, 266, 269, 350
Ceptaz, 92
Cerebral respiratory center, 347
Ceruloplasmin, 9
Chaddock's sign, 463
Charting, 470
Chest physiotherapy, 414
Children's dosages, 417
Chloramphenicol, 98
Chloramphenicol Sodium, 98
Chloride, 40
Chloride, serum, 9
Chloride, urine, 9
Chloromycetin Kapseals, 98
Chloromycetin Palmitate, 98
Chlorothiazide, 102
Chlorthalidone, 104
Cholesterol, 10, 43
Cholesterol HDL, 10
Cin-Quin, 192
Circulation, 418
Cirrhosis, 36, 44-46
Claforan, 88
Cleocin HCl, 100
Cleocin Phosphate, 100
Clindamycin HCl, 100
Clindamycin Phosphate, 100
Clonidine HCl, 106
Clotting factor, 446
Coarctation of the aorta (COA), 437
Coccidioidomycosis, 67
Cold agglutins, 10
Colloid oncotic pressure (COP), 48
Complement (C-3), 10
Complement (C-4), 10
Complement, total, 10
Complete blood count (CBC), 11
  Differential white cell count, 11
  Red blood cell count (RBC), 11
  White blood cell count (WBC), 11
  White blood cell differential, 34
Compliance (Cl), 352
Concentration, 426
Congenital, 433
Continuous positive airway pressure (CPAP), 357
Controlled mechanical ventilation (CMV), 355
Coopernail sign, 463
Cor Pulmonale, 311
Corrigan's pulse, 463
Corticotropin releasing hormone (CRH), 388
Counterpulsation, 333
CPK isoenzymes, 14
Crackles, 366
  Coarse, 366
  Fine, 366
  Medium, 366
Cranial nerves, 407
Creatine phospokinase (CPK, CK), 14
Creatinine, 44
Creatinine clearance, 14
Creatinine serum, 14
Creatinine, urine, 15
Cryptococcal meningitis, 128
Crystals, 39
Crystapen, 175
Cullen's sign, 464

The ICU Quick Reference 491

Cushing's syndrome, 40-44, 46-47, 376
Cytomegalovirus, 61

D

Darier's sign, 464
Decreased diffusion, 348
Deep tendon reflexes, 406
Defibrillation, 424
Dehydration, 430
Delbet's sign, 464
Deponit, 168
Deterioration, 413
Diabetes insipidus, 40, 42, 391
Diabetes mellitus, 41, 43-44, 46, 379
Diabetic acidosis, 42, 46
Diachlor, 102
Diastole, 336
Diastolic augmentation, 336
DIC profile, 34
Dicrotic notch, 336
Diflucan, 128
Digitalis toxicity, 312
Digoxin, 15, 108
Dilantin, 177
Dilantin capsules, 177
Dilantin level, 15
DiPhen, 177
Diphenylan Sodium, 177
Disopyramide, 110
Dispos-a-Med isoproterenol HCl, 139
Disseminated intravascular coagulopathy (DIC), 36, 47, 369
Diulo, 153
Diuretic, 124, 130, 153, 197, 205
Diuril, 102
Diuril Sodium, 102
Dobutamine (Inotrex), 426
Dobutamine HCl, 113

Dobutrex, 113
Dopamine (Intropin), 426
Dopamine HCl, 115
Dorendorf's sign, 464
Drug administration rates, 428
Duchenne's sign, 464
Duroziez's sign, 464
Dynamic compliance (Cdyn), 353
Dyrenium, 205
Dysrhythmias, 187

E

E-Base, 119
E-Mycin, 119
E.E.S. 400, 119
Edecrin, 124
Edecrin Sodium, 124
Edema, 102, 130, 205
Effer-K, 180
Egophony, 367
Einthoven's triangle, 303
Ejection fraction, 336
12 lead EKG, 295
EKG rhythm determination, 294
EKG wave patterns, 290
Electrolyte, 180
Electrolyte replacement, 81
Electrolytes
  Imbalances, 373
Electromagnetic interference, 319
Electromechanical dissociation (EMD), 238
Electrophysiologic study, 319
Emphysema, 368
Empyema, 175
Endocarditis, 86
Endocrine dysfunction, 376
Endocrine problems, 389
Endocrine system, 388

492 Index

Endotracheal tube, 330
Eosinophil count, 16
Eosinophils, 35
Epidural hematoma, 403
Epigastric, 445
Epinephrine, 51, 117, 237, 239-240 425
Epinephrine (Adrenalin), 426
Epinephrine infusion, 425
Epinephrine pediatric, 117
Epstein-Barr virus, 61
Erb's sign, 464-465
Ery-Tab, 119
Eryc, 119
Eryped, 119
Erythrocyte sedimentation rate (ESR), 16
Erythromycin, 119
Erythromycin Base, 119
Erythromycin Estolate, 119
Erythromycin Ethylsuccinate, 119
Erythromycin Filmtabs, 119
Esmolol HCl, 122
Estriol, 16
Ethacrynic acid, 124
Ethanol, 48
Ethmozine, 162
Euglobulin clot lysis, 16
Ewart's sign, 465
Expiratory reserve volume (ERV), 350
Eyes, 448-449

F

Face and scalp, 449
Facial nerve, 407
Farenheit, 441
Fat, fecal quantitative, 16
Fat, fecal, qualitative, 16
Febrile agglutinins, 16
Fibrin split products (FSP), 16
Fibrinogen, 17
Fick method, 261
Fixed rate pacing, 317
Flecainide acetate, 126
Fluconazole, 128
Folic acid, 17
Follicle-stimulating hormone, 388
Forced expiratory volume (FEV), 349
Forced vital capacity (FVC), 349
Fortaz, 92
Fumide, 130
Functional residual capacity (FRC), 350
Fungizone IV, 67
Furomide M.D., 130
Furosemide, 52, 130, 425

G

Gamma glutamyl transferase (GGT), 17
Gamman's sign, 465
Gangrene, 175
Garamycin, 132
Gastrointestinal, 471
Gen-K, 180
Genitourinary, 471
Gentamicin, 52
Gentamicin levels, 17
Gentamicin sulfate, 132
Glabella reflex, 465
Glasgow coma scale (GCS), 399
Globulin, 17
Globulin serum, total, 17
Glomerular filtration rate (GFR), 395
Glossopharyngeal nerve, 407
Glucose, 44, 425
Glucose, CSF, 18
Glucose, serum

Fasting, 18
Glucose, urine, 18
Glycosylated hemoglobin, 18
Gonorrhea, 175
Gram negative bacteria, 84, 92
Gram negative organisms, 86, 88, 90, 94, 137, 175, 201
Gram positive bacteria, 84, 92
Gram positive organisms, 86, 88, 90, 94, 137, 175, 201
Granular casts, 38
Grey Turner's sign, 268, 465
Guillain Barrè, 347

H

Ham's test, 18
Haptoglobin, 18
Head injury patients, 400
Heart block, 324
Heart rate calculation, 293
Heart sounds
    Auscultation of, 328
    Ejection clicks, 329
    Murmurs, 329
    S1, 328
    S2, 328
    S3, 328
    S4, 329
Hematocrit, (HCT), 12 47, 268
Hemocystine, 19
Hemodynamic monitoring, 174
Hemodynamic parameters
    Formulas and normals for, 257
Hemoglobin, 47, 268
    Mean corpuscular (MCH), 13
    Mean corpuscular concentration (MCHC), 13
Hemoglobin (HMG), 12
Hemoglobin F, 18

Hemolytic anemia, 45
Hemorrhage (subungual), 465
Hemosiderin, 18
Heparin, 35
Hepatitis, 45-46
Herpes
    Genital, 61-62
    Simplex, 61-62
Herpes I and II immunofluorescence titer, 19
Herpes simplex encephalitis, 61
Hill's sign, 465
Hirsutism, 377
Histamine, 35
Histiocytes, 35
HIV (human immunodeficiency virus), 128
Homan's sign, 465
Hoover sign, 466
Hyaline casts, 38
Hydralazine HCl, 134
Hygroton, 104
Hylidone, 104
Hyperalbuminemia, 34
Hyperaldosteronism, 40, 42, 205
Hypercalcemia, 33, 313, 373, 384
Hypercapnia, 354
Hyperchloremia, 385
Hyperglycemia, 373
Hyperkalemia, 81, 182, 312, 374, 382 383
Hypermagnesemia, 33, 81, 313, 375, 386
Hypernatremia, 33, 374, 381-382
Hyperparathyroidism, 40, 43
Hyperphosphatemia, 81, 375, 385
Hyperpituitarism, 44
Hypertension, 59, 102, 106, 130, 189, 378

Hyperthermia, 267
Hyperthyroidism, 40, 44
Hypertonic dehydration, 432
Hypertrophy, 309
Hyperventilation, 355
Hyperviscosity, 33
Hypoalbuminemia, 33
Hypocalcemia, 81, 373, 383-384
Hypochloremia, 385
Hypogastric, 446
Hypoglossal nerve, 407
Hypoglycemia, 373
Hypokalemia, 181, 312, 374, 382-383
Hypomagnesemia, 375, 384-385
Hyponatremia, 374, 380
Hypoparathyroidism, 41
Hypoperfusion, 370
Hypophosphatemia, 375, 386
Hypopituitarism, 379
Hypotension, 267, 378
Hypothalamus, 388
Hypothyroidism, 43, 45-46
Hypoventilation, 355
Hypoxemia, 267
Hypoxia, 370
Hyptomic dehydration, 431

I

Idiopathic hypertropic subaortic stenosis, 189
Ilosone, 119
Ilotycin Gluceptate, 119
Imipenem/cilastatin, 137
Immunoglobulin A (IgA), 19
Immunoglobulin E (IgE), 19
Immunoglobulin G (IgG), 20
Immunoglobulin G, CSF, 20
Immunoglobulin M (IgM), 20
Implantable pulse generator, 320

Impulse, 320
Inderal, 189
Inderal 10, 189
Inderal 20, 189
Inderal 40, 189
Inderal 60, 189
Inderal 80, 189
Inderal LA, 189
Indications for weaning from ventilator, 360
Indocin, 48
Infections, 84, 86, 88, 90, 92, 94, 119, 133, 137, 142, 201
Inocor, 70
Inspiratory capacity (IC), 349-350

Inspiratory reserve volume (IRV), 350
Intermittent mandatory ventilation (IMV), 356
Intra-aortic balloon pump (IABP), 333
Intra-aortic balloon therapy (IABP), 334, 335
Intropin, 115
Ipran, 189
Iron, 20
Iron-binding capacity (TIBC), 20
Isoproterenol (Isuprel), 426
Isoproterenol HCl, 139
Isoptin, 207
Isoptin SR, 207
Isovolumetric contraction, 336
Isovolumetric relaxation, 336
Isuprel, 139
Isuprel Glossets, 139
Isuprel Mistometer, 139

The ICU Quick Reference 495

J
Janeway's spots (lesions), 466
Jenamicin, 132
Jugular vein distention (JVD), 350

K
K-Lyte, 180
K-Lyte DS, 180
K-Lyte/Cl, 180
K-Tab, 180
Kanamycin sulfate, 142
Kantrex, 142
Kaochlor, 180
Kashiuda's sign, 466
Kay Ciel, 180
Kay-Dur, 180
Kaylixir, 180
Kefurox, 96
Kefzol, 86
Kehr's sign, 466
Kermig's sign, 466
Ketones, urine, 21
Kleist's sign, 466
Klor, 180
Klor-Con, 180
Klortrix, 180
Klorvess, 180
Kussmaul's sign, 269, 466

L
LA line
    Discontinuing, 264
LA pressures
    Diastolic, 264
    Mean, 264
    Systolic, 264
Labetalol, 144
Laboratory findings
    Suggestive of medical disorders, 40
Lactic acid, serum, 21
Lactic dehydrogenase (LDH), 22, 45
Lanoxin, 108
Lasix, 130
LDH isoenzymes, 22
LE Prep, 22
Lead, 320
    Atrial, 320
    Endocardial, 320
    Low threshold, 320
    Myocardial, 320
    Permanent, 320
    Steroid eluting, 320
    Temporary, 321
    Transvenous, 321
    Ventricular, 321
Lead active fixation, 320
Leads, 286
    Placement of, 286
Lee White clotting time, 22
Left anterior hemiblock, 310
Left atrial (LA) lines, 263
Left atrial abnormality, 307
Left atrial line, 331
Left atrial pressure, 258
Left atrial pressure waveforms, 263
Left axis deviation, 304
Left bundle branch block, 310
Left hypochondriac, 445
Left iliac, 446
Left lumbar, 445
Left posterior hemiblock, 311
Left ventricular hypertrophy, 308
Left ventricular stroke work index (LVSWI), 258
Leichtenstern's sign, 467
Less severe infections, 87

496 Index

Level of consciousness, 269
Levophed, 173
Lewis lead, 286
Lhermitte's sign, 467
Lidocaine, 237
Lidocaine (Xylocaine), 425-426
Lidocaine HCl, 146
Lidocaine level, 23
Lidopen Auto-Injector, 146
Limb leads, 295
Lipase, serum, 23
Lithium level, 23
Liver disease, 130
Loniten, 160
Loop diuretic, 79
Lopressor, 155
Lumbar puncture, 414
Luramide, 130
Lymphocytes, 35

M

Macewan's sign, 467
Magnesium, 40
   Daily approximate requirements, 376
Magnesium replenishers, 149
Magnesium serum, 23
Magnesium sulfate, 149, 237
Mandol, 84
Mannitol (Osmitrol), 425
Mastoiditis, 175
Maximum inspiratory pressure (MIP), 349
Mean arterial pressure (MAP), 259, 336
Mean corpuscular volume (MCV), 13
Mechanical ventilation, 355
Mediastinal chest tube, 340
Mediastinal chest tubes, 332

Medication, 426
Medihaler-Iso, 139
Mefoxin, 90
Membrane potential, 321
Meningitis, 67, 92, 94, 175
Metabolic acidosis, 33-34, 195
Metacytes, 35
Methadopa, 151
Methyldopa/Methyldopate HCl, 151
Metolazone, 153
Metoprolol, 155
Mexiletine HCl, 158
Mexitil, 158
Micro-K, 180
Microsomal antibody titer, 23
Migraines, 189
Minipress, 183
Minitran, 168
Minodyl, 160
Minoxidil, 160
Minute ventilation (VE), 349
Minute volume (VE), 349
Modified chest lead, 287
Monitan, 59
Monocytes, 35
Monotest, 23
Moricizine, 162
Morphine, 164, 425
Mucocutaneous leishmaniasis, 67
Murphy's sign, 467
Musculoskeletal, 472
Myelocytes, 35
Myeloma, 33
Mykrox, 153
Myocardial infarction, 333
   EKG changes in, 306
Myxedema coma, 379

The ICU Quick Reference 497

N

Nadolol, 166
Naloxone (Narcan), 425
Narcotic analgesic, 164
Nasal cannula, 347
Nasogastric tube, 332
NBG code, 321
Negative inspiratory force (NIF), 349
Nephrotic syndrome, 46, 130
Nervous system, 452
Neurologic, 471
Neutrophils, 34
Niacinamide, 51
Nicoladoni's sign, 467
Nipride, 171
Nitro-Bid, 168
Nitro-Bid IV, 168
Nitro-Bid Plateau Caps, 168
Nitro-Dur, 168
Nitroblue tetrazolium titer (NBT), 23
Nitrocine Timecaps, 168
Nitrodisc, 168
Nitrogard, 168
Nitroglycerin, 168, 426
Nitroglyn, 168
Nitrol, 168
Nitrong, 168
Nitropress, 171
Nitroprusside sodium, 171
Nitrostat, 168
Non-competitive pacing, 317
Norepinephrine bitartrate, 173
Norisoprine Aerotrol, 139
Normal laboratory values, 3
Normodyne, 144
Norpace CR, 110
Novospiroton, 197

O

Obtundation, coma, 452
Occult blood, fecal, 24
Occult blood, urine, 24
Oculocardiac reflex, 467
Oculomotor nerve, 407
Olfactory nerve, 407
Optic nerve, 407
Orbicularis sign, 468
Oropharyngeal candidiasis, 128
Orosomucoid, 24
Osmolality, serum, 24
Osmolality, urine, 24
Osmotic fragility, 24
Osteomyelitis, 175
Overdrive pacing, 321
Oversensing, 321
Ox-cell hemolysis titer, 24
Oxygen delivery, 347
Oxygen dissociation curve, 367
Oxygen therapy, 351
Oxygen toxicity, 351-352
Oxygen transport, 352

P

P wave, 263, 292
PA catheter waveforms, 263
PA monitors, 277
Pacemaker
   A-V interval, 318
   A-V sequential, 322
   A-V universal, 322
   Artificial, 321
   Asynchronous, 322
   Atrial synchronous, 322
   Atrial tracking, 318
   Blanking period, 318
   Burst pacing, 318

498 Index

Capture, 318
Connections, 331
Demand, 322
Dual chamber pacing, 319
Electrogram, 319
End of life, 319
Escape interval, 319
Exit block, 319
Fusion beat, 319
Hysteresis, 319
Impedance, 320
Rate responsive, 322
Sensing threshold, 323
Troubleshooting, 326
Underdrive pacing, 323
Undersensing, 323
Pacemaker terminology, 317
Pacemakers, 315
   Action potential, 317
   Basic parts of, 315
Pacer reject, 337
Pacing stimuli, 324
Pancreas, 389
Pancreatitis, 36, 45-46
Pancuronium (Pavulon), 425
Parathyroid gland, 389
Partial thromboplastin time (PTT), 25
Pastia's sign, 468
Patent ductus arteriosus (PDA), 435
Peak inspiratory pressure, 350
Pectoriloquy, 367
Pediatric coma scale, 401
Pediatric emergency medication, 424
Penicillin G sodium, 175
Pentacef, 92
Percutaneous transluminal coronary angioplast, 341
Perez's reflex, 468
Perez's sign, 468

Peripheral resistance, 70
Peritonitis, 84
Persantine, 48
pH, urine, 24
Phencyclidine (PCP), 454
Phenobarbital level, 25
Phenytoin level, 25
Phenytoin Oral Suspension, 177
Phenytoin sodium, 177
Pheochromocytoma, 44, 47, 189, 378
Phlebostatic axis, 276, 280
Phosphate, 41
Phosphorus, serum, 25
Phosphorus, urine, 26
Piotrowski's sign, 468
Pitres's sign, 468
Pituitary gland, 388
Pituitary glands
   Anterior pituitary, 388
   Posterior pituitary, 388
Plasma hemoglobin, 26
Plasminogen, 26
Plateau pressure, 350
Platelet count, 13, 26
Platelets, 48
Pleural chest tubes, 332
Pleural friction rub, 366
Pneumonia, 175
Pneumothorax, 358
Polycythemia, 47
Positive End Expiratory Pressure (PEEP), 356-357
Potachlor, 180
Potage, 180
Potain's sign, 468
Potasalan, 180
Potassium, 41, 180
   Daily approximate requirements, 376

The ICU Quick Reference 499

Potassium Chloride, 180, 425
Potassium Gluconate, 180
Potassium, serum, 26
Potassium, urine, 26
PR interval, 292
Prazosin HCl, 183
Prealbumin, 26
Precordial chest leads, 295
Preload, 254, 337
Premature ventricular contractions, 295
Pressure limit, 360
Pressure support ventilation (PSV), 356
Prevost's sign, 469
Primaxin IV, 137
Procainamide, 184, 237
Procainamide HCl, 184
Procainamide level, 27
Procan SR, 184
Promine, 184
Pronestyl, 184
Propafenone, 187
Propranolol, 189
Propranolol HCl, 189
Propranolol Intensol, 189
Protein, total serum, 27
Protein, total, urine, 27
Prothrombin time (PT), 27
Pseudocholinesterase, 27
Pulmonary artery, 265, 274
Pulmonary artery catheter, 274
Pulmonary artery line, 331
Pulmonary artery pressure (PAP), 350
Pulmonary artery pressures, 355
    Diastolic, 275
    Mean, 275
    Systolic, 275
Pulmonary capillary wedge pressure (PCWP), 70, 265-266, 269, 275, 350
Pulmonary edema, 130
Pulmonary embolism, 311
Pulmonary hypertension, 311
Pulmonary vascular resistance (PVR), 257
Pulmonary vascular resistance index (PVRI), 258
Pulmonic valve, 265
Pulseless electrical activity, 238

Q

Q wave, 292
Q waves, 343
QRS complex, 287, 290
QRS duration, 292
Q-T interval, 292
Quinadine Gluconate, 192
Quinalan, 192
Quincke's pulse, 469
Quinidine, 48, 192
Quinidine level, 28
Quinidine Sulfate, 192
Quinquaud's sign, 469

R

R wave, 292
Rapid ventricular ejection phase, 337
Rate, 349
Red blood cell casts, 39
Red blood cells, 37, 47
Red cell width distribution (RDW), 13
Reducing substances, fecal and urine, 28
Refractory period, 337
Renal failure
    Post renal, 394

500 Index

Pre-renal, 394
Renin-angiotensin aldosterone feedback system, 379
Residual volume (RV), 349
Respiratory equations, 352
Respiratory synctial virus antibodies (RSV), 28
Reticulocyte count, 28
Retroperitoneal bleeding, 268
Reye's syndrome, 44
Rheumatoid factor (RA), 27
Rhythmin, 184
Right atrial abnormality, 307
Right atrial pressure (RA) waveforms, 265
Right atrium, 265, 274
Right axis deviation, 304
Right bundle branch block, 310
Right hypochondriac, 445
Right iliac, 446
Right lumber, 445
Right ventricle, 265
Right ventricular (RV) pressure, 258
Right ventricular hypertrophy, 307
Right ventricular stroke work index (RVSWI), 259
Rocephin, 94
Rogaine, 160
Rotch's sign, 469
Roth's spots, 469
Roxanol, 164
Roxanol 100, 164
Roxanol Rescudose, 164
Roxanol SR, 164
rs pattern, 287
Rumpel-Leed's sign, 469
Rythmol, 187

S

Safety chamber, 337
Salicylate level, 28
Salicylate toxicity, 42
Sectral, 59
Sedation, 414
Sedimentation rate, 29
Septicemia, 86, 88, 94
Serotinin 5HIAA quantitative, 29
Serum glutamic-oxaloascetic transaminase, 46
Serum osmolality, 48
Severe infections, 89, 91
SGOT, 29
SGPT, 29
Shift to the left, 367
Shift to the right, 367
Shock, 44
    Anaphylactic, 267
    Cardiogenic, 266
    Neurogenic, 268
    Septic, 267
    States of, 266
    Three stages of, 269
Shunting, 353
SIADH, 376, 392
Sibilant wheezes, 366
Signorelli's sign, 469
Sincomen, 197
Sinus arrest, 75
Sinus tachycardia, 59
Skin, 471
Skin and mucous membranes, 450-451
Slow-K, 180
Sodium, 42
    Daily approximate requirements, 376
Sodium bicarbonate, 195, 239

The ICU Quick Reference 501

Sodium Nitroprusside (nipride), 171, 426
Sodium, serum, 30
Sodium, urine, 30
Sonorous wheezes, 366
Specific gravity
   Urine, 30
Spinal accessory nerve, 407
Spironolactone, 197
Sporotrichosis, 67
Squamous epithelial cells, 38
Static compliance, 353
Stroke volume (SV), 257, 337
Stroke volume index (SVI), 258
Sub-Quin, 184
Subarachnoid hematoma, 404
Subclavian arteries, 334
Subdural hematoma, 403
Suctioning, 413
Sugar water test, 30
Suprasystolic augmentation, 337
Surgical prophylaxis, 86
Sweat chloride, 30
Symptomatic bradycardias, 75
Symptoms and possible poisons, 448
Syphilis, serological test, 29
Systemic vascular resistance (SVR), 70, 258, 266, 267, 337, 350
Systemic vascular resistance index (SVRI), 258
Systole, 314, 337

T

T wave, 263, 343
T waves, 313
Tachycardia, 267, 294, 378, 458
Tachycardias, 64
Tachydysrhythmias, 59
Tachypnea, 370

Tambocor, 126
Tazicef, 92
Tazidime, 92
Temperature equivalents, 441
Temporary pacing
   Indications for, 324
Tenormin, 72
Tension pneumothorax, 350
Tetanus, 175
Tetralogy of Fallot, 436
Thalitone, 104
Theophylline level, 31
Threshold, 337
Thrombin clotting time, 31
Thromboplastin, 31
Thyroid crisis, 389
Thyroid gland, 389
Thyroid-stimulating hormone (TSH), 31, 388
Thyrotoxicosis, 377, 379
Ticar, 201
Ticarcillin disodium, 201
Ticaripen, 201
Tidal volume (VT), 349
Timentin, 201
Timing, 337
Timolol, 199
Timolol maleate, 199
Tobramycin level, 32
Tocainide HCl, 203
Tonocard, 203
Tonsillar (medullary) herniation, 405
Total lung capacity (TLC), 350
Total peripheral resistance (TPR), 258
Total protein, 46
Toxicity, 81
Tracheal mask, 347
Trandate, 144
Transferrin level, 32

Tremors, 190
Tri-K, 180
Triamterene, 205
Tricuspid valve, 265
Tridil, 168
Trigeminal nerve, 407
Trigger, 337
Triglycerides, 32
Trochlear nerve, 407
Twin-K, 180

U

Ulcerative colitis, 40, 46
Umbilical, 445
Unassisted aortic end-diastolic pressure, 338
Unassisted systole (UAS), 338
Uncal (tentorial) herniation, 404
Uric acid, 32
Urinary candidiasis, 128
Urinary output, 331
Urine
    Microscopic examination of, 37

V

V wave, 263, 265, 314
Vagus nerve, 407
Vanillylmandelic acid (VMA), 33
Varicella-zoster virus, 61
Vascular resistance, 70
Vein sign, 470
Ventilator modes, 355
Ventilators, 359
Ventricles, 314
Ventricular ectopy, 279
Ventricular fibrillation, 195, 233, 235
Ventricular filling, 338

Ventricular pressure, 265
Ventricular tachycardia, 195, 233, 235
Venturi mask, 347
Verapamil HCl, 207
Verelan, 207
Vital capacity (VC), 349-350
Vitamin D deficiency, 81
Voice sounds, 366

W

Wheezes, 366
White blood cell casts, 38
White blood cells, 37
Wolff-Parkinson-White (WPW) syndrome, 342

X

x Descent, 265
Xylocaine HCl, 146

Y

y Descent, 265
Yeast, 39

Z

Zaroxolyn, 153
Zinacef, 96
Zolicef, 86
Zovirax, 61

Skidmore-Roth Publishing, Inc. Order Form
1(800) 825-3150

Qty.	Title	Price	Total
	Drug Comparison Handbook, 2nd ed.	$29.95	
	1995 Nurse's Trivia Calendar	$9.95	
	RN NCLEX Review Cards, 2nd ed.	$24.95	
	PN/VN Review Cards	$24.95	
	Nurse's Survival Guide, 2nd ed.	$24.95	
	The Body in Brief, 2nd ed.	$26.95	
	The Obstetric Survival Guide	$24.95	
	The OBRA Guidelines for Quality Improvement in Long Term Care	$59.95	
	Diagnostic & Laboratory Cards, 2nd ed.	$23.95	
Tax of 8.25% applies to Texas residents only. UPS ground shipping $5 for first item, $1 each additional item.		Subtotal	

	8.25% Tax	
		Shipping
		TOTAL

Name	
Company	
Address	
City	
State	Zip
Phone	
___ Check enclosed ___ Visa ___ MasterCard	
Credit Card Number	
Card Holder Name	
Signature	Expiration Date

For fastest service call, 1-800-825-3150 or fax your order to us at (915) 877-4424. Orders are accepted by mail. Prices subject to change without notice.

Skidmore-Roth Publishing, Inc.
7730 Trade Center Avenue
El Paso, TX 79912